SPICE IT UP WITH ROBUST FLAVOR

DELICIOUS RECIPES

FOR LIFETIME WELLNESS

Digna I Cassens, MHA, RDN, CLT, FAND

First Edition, November 2017

This recipe book is a collection of original recipes I developed for my clients and my personal use.

Published by:
Cassens Associates – Diversified Nutrition Management Systems
558 Tahoe Avenue Yucca
Valley, CA 92284
dignacassens@gmail.com
http://flavorfulfortifiedfood.com

ISBN-10:0998143006
ISBN-13:978-0998143002

Printed and manufactured in the United States of America
First Printing: 2017 Cassens Associates
http://www.nutritionmanagementsystems.org

Table of Contents

To my mother Marina Martínez de Irizarry (1917 - 2014) who inspired me to create wholesome food and serve it with love.

This book not complete without stating my thanks and appreciation to my husband, who is always willing to taste new recipes and contribute candid opinions. His patience and support encourage me to continue my efforts and realize my dreams.

Digna I Cassens

About Me

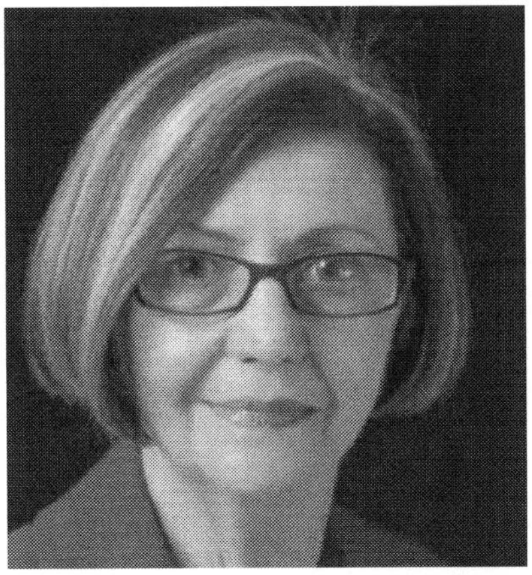

Digna Cassens, MHA, RDN, CLT, FAND

I'm a registered dietitian nutritionist (RDN), owner of a micro-practice, Diversified Nutrition Management System. I have a BS in Foods & Nutrition and completed a dietetic internship, a Master's degree in Healthcare Administration and have lifetime teaching credentials for Community Colleges in California. As a Certified LEAP Therapist I treat clients with food sensitivities as well as chronic diseases, weight issues and allergies. I'm very active in the Academy of Nutrition and Dietetics (AND) and belong to several practice groups contributing as a volunteer member of various committees. During my long-years in the profession I've received many honors, such as the 2014 Distinguished Member Award from Dietetics in Healthcare Communities (DHCC) and the 2015 Excellence in Communication, Consulting and Private Practice Award from the California Academy of Nutrition and Dietetics.

I launched my company in 2011 after many decades in the corporate world. I now limit my practice to consulting for homes for adults with intellectual and physical disabilities and assisted living centers. I also continue to provide nutrition and wellness counseling to individuals and groups and occasionally accept speaking engagements. Currently I live with my husband, 3 rescued dogs, a cat and rescued water turtles in the Mohave Desert area in Southern California, spending much of my time creating healthy nutritious food and writing recipe books.

My publications include *Flavorful Fortified Food – Recipes to Enrich your Life, Food First - Enhancing the Quality of Life using Fortified Food, Dining Services Policies and Procedures Manuals for Long-Term Care Communities, Food for Group Homes, Simplified Diets and Nutrition Guidelines, Dining Services Orientation and Training for Cooks and Dining Services Education & Training Manual.*

Connect with me and get to know me better.

http://www.facebook.com/cassensassociates, http://www.nutritionmanagementsystems.org, https://twitter.com/@dithisland, https://www.pinterest.com/digtheisland, https://www.linkedin.com/in/digna-cassens-mha-rdn-clt

PREFACE

I invite you to enjoy tasty food that is also stress free to prepare. Relax knowing you don't have to be an experienced cook or have a gourmet kitchen to achieve delicious results with these simplified recipes. With a few herbs and spices you can change a boring meal into a remarkable one.

These nutritious recipes, packed with *robust* flavor, are so easy and affordable! This is "scratch" cooking at its best, avoiding processed ingredients and giving you choices according to your time and skills. Only you will ever know these dishes are moderate in sodium, fat and calories!

I wrote this book because of my love for cooking and eating good food; the recipes are reflective of the way I cook. I like flavorful food that I can prepare quickly and have very little cleanup afterwards. My friends and family know that they can drop in any time and have a meal fit for kings in a couple of hours. Being a food aficionado and loving to eat I like interesting food with layers of flavor; mouth- watering food.

I've enjoyed a long career in nutrition as a registered dietitian nutritionist providing consulting services to long-term care communities and private individuals, some chronically ill and confined to their homes. The experience helped me realize the need for simplified recipes, so I started sharing recipes with the clients and their care givers during my visits. Starting the visits discussing food and sharing a couple of healthy recipes always received a positive response. I was able to adapt their favorite recipes to healthier versions, or make a few seasoning changes to mine to suit their taste.

The 80 recipes in this book include basic nutrition information and are moderate in fat, sodium and sugar. The nutrient analysis includes calories, fat, protein, carbohydrate, dietary fiber, cholesterol, sugars, sodium and diabetic exchanges, proving once more that it's possible to eat very healthy food that is delicious. All ingredients are commonly found in the local markets and your own cupboards.

ABOUT THIS BOOK

Organization

- There are 80 recipes grouped by categories; Appetizers & Light Snacks, Bakery & Desert, Beverages, Breakfasts, Entrées, and Sauces, Seasonings & Soups.
- The Table of Contents lists categories and recipes in alphabetical order. For ease in finding recipes there is also an alpha-numerical index included in the last pages.
- Although the easiest way to find a recipe is alphabetically under each category, for your convenience page numbers are also included on the page lower margin.

Nutritional Analysis

- The nutritional analysis is provided as a guide and calculated using the Master Cook 15 (*http://www.mastercook.com*) nutrient data sourced from the USDA data base and manufacturers information for their products.
- Some nutrient values may vary based on brand and the nutrient data used by the manufacturers.
- Optional items, variations and garnishes are not included in the nutritional analysis.

Portions

Recipes do not take into consideration variations in appetites. If you need to serve larger portions or serve more people it's easy to increase amount you're making.

- When the portion size is the same, recipe conversion factors are determined by taking the number of portions you want and divide by the number of portions you have in the recipe. For example, you want 15 portions. By using the 6 portion information on the recipe (15 ÷ 6), your conversion factor is 2.5. This means you multiple each ingredient by 2.5 to determine the quantity of each ingredient. If you have 6 portions and want 4 portions (4 ÷ 6), your conversion factor is 0.66. This means you multiply each ingredient by 0.66 to determine the quantity of each ingredient needed.
- As yields (number of portions) are increased or decreased the cooking time for some recipes might change.

There is no love sincerer than the love of food.

George Bernard Shaw, *Man and Superman*

Appetizers
Light Snacks

Corn Coconut Chutney

A delicious blend of blackened corn, pepper and spices with a touch of the tropics

Yield: 1 1/2 quarts

Preparation Time: 45 minutes

Ingredients

6 cups corn kernels, frozen, canned or fresh
1/2 Tablespoon olive oil, or may use avocado oil for a lighter taste
1 Cup diced red bell pepper
1 Cup diced green bell pepper
1/2 Cup Jalapeño Chile Pepper, seeded and minced
1 1/2 Cups red onion, diced
1 Cup Crushed Pineapple, juice packed
1 Tablespoon black pepper, more or less to taste
1 Tablespoon Cayenne, more or less to taste
2 Teaspoons kosher salt, more or less to taste
1 1/2 Cups coconut cream, canned, unsweetened
1 Tablespoon Lemon Juice

Method

In a large skillet heat oil, add drained corn kernels and stir fry until golden

Add onions & diced peppers and continue stir frying to cook peppers until just tender but still crisp

Add salt, black pepper & Cayenne, stir to mix seasonings in

Add crushed pineapple and coconut cream. Cover and simmer on low heat for 15 minutes

Add lemon juice and stir to mix. Refrigerate until needed and serve either hot or cold.

Servings: 24

Per Serving (excluding unknown items): 86 Calories; 4g Fat (36.1% calories from fat); 2g Protein; 13g Carbohydrate; 2g Dietary Fiber; 0mg Cholesterol; 169mg Sodium. Exchanges: 1/2 Grain(Starch); 1/2 Vegetable; 0 Fruit; 1/2 Fat.

Crispy Potato Skins

If not stuffing the potato skin shells use the leftover pulp as follows:
1- Add your choice of salt, pepper, sliced green onion, crumbled bacon, shredded cheese and/or fresh herbs. Top with bread crumbs, dot with butter and bake until heated through.
2- Sauté chopped onion in butter until tender. Stir in potatoes and continue to cook and stir until heated through.
3- Make a potato salad using warm potato insides. Toss with bottled vinaigrette dressing or mayonnaise, sliced green onion, chopped olives and crumbled bacon. Chill.
4- Add to soups to thicken them.
A hearty appetizer, light lunch or dinner side dish.

Ingredients
4 medium potatoes (about 2 lbs.)
1 Tablespoon Olive Oil
1 Tablespoon Melted Butter
1/8 Teaspoon salt
1 Teaspoon pepper, or to taste
1 Teaspoon chili powder
1/4 Cup Grated Parmesan Cheese
Serving Ideas: Serve 2 stuffed shells per serving with a side of salsa, low fat yogurt or low fat Ranch dressing.

Servings: 8

Method

Preheat oven to 400°F. Scrub potatoes & bake for 45 minutes to 1 hour or until tender.

Cut each potato lengthwise into 4 quarters. Scoop potato pulp from skins leaving a 1/2" thick layer of potato. Save pulp.

Brush skins inside and out with melted butter. Sprinkle with salt and pepper.

Place skins, skin-side down, on a baking sheet. Bake about 15 minutes or until crisp. Sprinkle with Parmesan cheese. Serve hot. Serve 2 skins per serving.

In the meantime, coarsely mash pulp, add butter and seasonings and toss to mix well.

Remove skins and turn them over. Lower oven temperature to 300°F and stuff the skins with the mashed and seasoned pulp.

Return to the oven and reheat for 10 minutes. Remove from oven and sprinkle with Parmesan cheese.

Sprinkle with Parmesan cheese.

Per Serving (excluding unknown items): 89 Calories; 4g Fat (39.5% calories from fat); 2g Protein; 11g Carbohydrate; 1g Dietary Fiber; 6mg Cholesterol; 111mg Sodium. Exchanges: 1 Grain(Starch); 0 Lean Meat; 1/2 Fat.

Deli Bagel Pizza Bites

1) These small bagel pizzas are a great snack or appetizer.
2) If you find small mini-bagels you can use these instead; just slice in half instead of quarters.
A healthy appetizer or light snack

Yield: 1/4 Bagel Each

Ingredients

6 Each rye or pumpernickel bagels, quartered, split and toasted lightly
1 Cup marinara sauce
1/3 Pound thinly sliced turkey pastrami
1/3 Pound thinly sliced low fat Swiss cheese
1/3 Pound ham
Serving Ideas: 1 - May use English muffins cut in quarters instead of bagels

Servings: 12

Preparation Time: 25 minutes

Method

Preheat oven to 375° F.

Cut bagels in quarters crosswise then separate top and bottom sections

Place in baking sheet and toast slightly

Place 1 teaspoon pizza sauce on to each piece, top with diced pastrami, ham, and cheese slices

Bake for 10 minutes until cheese melts.

Heat any remaining sauce and use as extra topping or for dipping

Per Serving (excluding unknown items): 249 Calories; 10g Fat (35.3% calories from fat); 13g Protein; 27g Carbohydrate;1g Dietary Fiber; 30mg Cholesterol; 677mg Sodium. Exchanges: 1 1/2 Grain(Starch); 1 Lean Meat; 1 Fat; 0 Other Carbohydrates.

Hummus Dip

1. Garnish with chopped parsley and/or oregano.
2. Mint leaves add an unexpected and refreshing kick.
Add the ingredients in the order listed. It's important.

Yield: 2 cups

Ingredients

2 Tablespoons Tahini
2 Tablespoons Lemon juice, or more to taste
2 Tablespoons olive oil
1 Clove garlic, large - or 1 teaspoon crushed or minced garlic (or more garlic to taste)
16 Ounces canned chickpeas, garbanzos
1 Dash kosher salt, about 1/8 tsp
1/8 Dash white pepper, about 1/8 tsp
3 Tablespoons water, add a bit more water as desired
2 Tablespoons olive oil, in addition to adding to mixture use to top before serving
2 Tablespoons paprika, sprinkle on top before serving
Serving Ideas: 1- Serve with pita bread strips or wedges, toasted pita bread or chips, crackers, bread sticks, toast, or vegetables for dipping
2- May omit Tahini for a less nutty, less creamy product and increase olive oil by 2 Tbsp
3- For a smokier flavor add paprika to the mixture when processing then add on top again as garnish

Method

In food processor combine tahini & lemon juice. Process to mix to a creamy state. Scrape sides and process again if needed

Add olive oil, crushed garlic and cumin, process to mix scraping sides as needed to mix

Drain garbanzos, rinse with water and shake dry.

Add half of the garbanzos into processor with the Tahini mixture and process for 1 - 2 minutes, scraping sides if needed.

Add remaining half of garbanzos and process for 2 - 3 minutes.

Taste and adjust salt and pepper as needed

If not smooth enough process until it's a creamy paste. if too thick add 2 - 3 tablespoons water.

Place into serving bowl. Pour olive oil and sprinkle with paprika.

Serve with pita chips or pita bread wedges or as a vegetable dip.

Servings: 16

Per Serving (excluding unknown items): 78 Calories; 5g Fat (53.6% calories from fat); 2g Protein; 8g Carbohydrate; 2g Dietary Fiber; 0mg Cholesterol; 102mg Sodium. Exchanges: 1/2 Grain(Starch); 0 Lean Meat; 0 Vegetable; 0 Fruit; 1 Fat.

Mini Rice Crackers Appetizer

Deli meats served on a crisp rice cake - an Asian-Italian fusion perfect as a light snack or appetizer
The bag has 25 rice cake thins, but since they're so crunchy I know you're going to bite into one as soon as you open the bag! So the recipe is for 24.

Yield: 24 servings

Ingredients
24 Each Rice Cake Thins
1/3 Cup marinara sauce
3 Ounces Pastrami Slices, cut into 4 pieces
3 Slices Mozzarella Cheese, cut into 4 pieces
3 Slices Turkey Breast Slices, cut into 4 pieces

Servings: 24

Preparation Time: 25 minutes

Method

Preheat oven to 375° F.

Place rice cakes on baking sheet.

Spoon about 1 teaspoon sauce onto each bagel half.

Cut each deli meat into fourths; straight down the middle, then crosswise

Layer deli meat quarters on top ending with cheese on top

Finish off with a dollop of sauce or sour cream

Bake 5 minutes or until cheese melts.

Per Serving (excluding unknown items): 315 Calories; 6g Fat (18.7% calories from fat); 15g Protein; 48g Carbohydrate;2g Dietary Fiber; 17mg Cholesterol; 607mg Sodium. Exchanges: 3 Grain(Starch); 1/2 Lean Meat; 1 Fat; 0 Other Carbohydrates.

Spicy Cream Cheese Spread on Toast Points

Don't limit yourself to toast points; this delicious spread goes well with vegetables too

Ingredients
2 Packages 8 Ounce Packages Cream Cheese
1/4 Cup Butter, softened not melted
1 Tablespoon Dijon Mustard
1/2 Cup Mayonnaise
1 Tablespoon Garlic Powder
2 Teaspoons Pepper
1 Teaspoon Cayenne Pepper
1/4 Cup Grated Parmesan Cheese
1/4 Cup Tablespoon Dry White Wine
1/4 Cup Minced Fresh Parsley
6 Slices Whole Wheat Bread, cut in 4 diagonally & toasted lightly
Serving Ideas: 1- Spread on toast points or crackers
2- Slice celery diagonally into 3 inch pieces and stuff with softened cheese; refrigerate until using
3 -Serve as a spread or dip and let everyone serve themselves

Preparation Time: 30 minutes

Method

Soften cream cheese & butter

In a mixer whip all ingredients together

Chill before spreading on toast points, crackers or celery

May also use as a dip

Servings: 24

Per Serving (excluding unknown items): 73 Calories; 6g Fat (74.3% calories from fat); 1g Protein; 4g Carbohydrate; 1g Dietary Fiber; 7mg Cholesterol; 106mg Sodium. Exchanges: 0 Grain(Starch); 0 Lean Meat; 0 Vegetable; 1 Fat; 0 Other Carbohydrates.

Zucchini Bites

A nutritious munchie to serve any time; try as a snack, a light lunch with a bowl of soup or fresh salad, or serve as an appetizer for your next party

Ingredients
24 Each Zucchini Slices
1 Teaspoon Kosher Salt
1 Teaspoon Pepper
1 Tablespoon Olive Oil, extra virgin
12 Each Mozzarella Cheese Substitute Slices, cut in quarters
1 Cup Parmesan Cheese, grated
Serving Ideas: 1- For a less nutritious option the same toppings can be used on round crackers. Skip the salt and olive oil when substituting crackers

Servings: 12

Method

Slice zucchini in about 1/4 inch slices - the amount of zucchini needed depends on their size

Sprinkle each slice lightly with salt & pepper to help bring out the flavors

Drizzle olive oil on each slice to coat nicely but not soak

Top with 2 quartered slices of Mozzarella then sprinkle about 1 teaspoon Parmesan cheese on each

Bake in 300° oven for 5 - 10 minutes until cheeses melt. Leave the vegetable crunchy so it can be picked up like crackers

Per Serving (excluding unknown items): 113 Calories; 7g Fat (51.8% calories from fat); 6g Protein; 8g Carbohydrate; trace Dietary Fiber; 5mg Cholesterol; 473mg Sodium. Exchanges: 0 Grain(Starch); 1 Lean Meat; 0 Vegetable; 1 Fat; 1/2 Other Carbohydrates.

Bakery

&

Desserts

Easy Morning Fruit Muffins

A great breakfast or any time snack. High in fiber and moderate in calories. If using Old Fashioned oats soak in water/oil/egg mixture, if using Quick Cooking mix with cake mix & proceed

Yield: 24 medium

Ingredients

1/2 Cup Applesauce, Unsweetened
1/2 Cup Mashed Banana
1/4 Cup Diced Pear, or substitute any other berries
1/4 Cup Chopped Apple
1 Cup water
1/2 Cup Vegetable Oil
1 1/2 Cups oatmeal
1 Teaspoon cinnamon, or may use another preferred spice
1 Envelope cake mix, we used Duncan Hines vanilla, white or yellow cake mix
1/4 Cup Nuts, use almonds, pecans and walnuts

Servings: 24

Preparation Time: 15 minutes
Start to Finish Time: 1 hour
Method

Preheat oven to 325°F. Insert muffin liners into the tins.

In a large bowl mix water, oil, egg mixture and mix at low speed. If using Old Fashioned Oatmeal add, stir to mix and soak for 30 minutes. If using Quick Cooking add with cake mix and proceed.

Add cake mix beating at low speed for 1 minute, then at high speed for 2 to 3 minutes. Do not overmix

Mix in applesauce, mashed banana, diced pear and apple

Add flour & oatmeal mixture to wet ingredients. Stir gently until combined. Do not overmix and do not beat.

Add chopped nuts. Fold in gently. Do not overmix

TO BAKE

Measure batter into each muffin bowl filling about 3/4 full. Do not overfill or muffins will rise and overflow out of the pan making it difficult to remove without breaking once baked.

Bake for 15 - 20 minutes or until light brown. Muffin tops will look a bit cracked.

Cool before serving or may eat them hot topped with favorite fruit spread or peanut butter for an extra kick.

Muffins freeze well if tightly sealed. Thaw at room temperature and warm in microwave or toaster oven.

Per Serving (excluding unknown items): 141 Calories; 7g Fat (46.1% calories from fat); 2g Protein; 18g Carbohydrate; 1g Dietary Fiber; 0mg Cholesterol; 100mg Sodium. Exchanges: 0 Grain(Starch); 0 Lean Meat; 0 Fruit; 1 1/2 Fat; 1 Other Carbohydrates.

Easy Morning Spice Muffins

A great breakfast or any time snack and no one needs to know you started with a mix. High in fiber and moderate in calories.

1) We used Duncan Hines spice cake mix

2) If using Old Fashioned oatmeal mix in water/oil/egg mixture, if using Quick Cooking add to cake mix & proceed without soaking

Yield: 24 medium

Ingredients

1 Each banana, mashed in the bowl
1 Cup water
1/2 Cup Vegetable Oil
1 Cup oatmeal
1 Envelope cake mix
1 Teaspoon Cinnamon
1 Teaspoon Nutmeg
2 Teaspoons Ginger
1 Teaspoon Ground Clove
1 Teaspoon Cardamom
1/2 Cup walnuts
1/2 Cup dried cranberries, or may substitute raisins, cherries, blueberries

Serving Ideas: 1- To serve as a dessert top with chocolate chips while hot so they melt
2- Spread with slightly sweetened soft cream cheese

Servings: 24

Preparation Time: 30 minutes
Start to Finish Time: 1 hour

Method

Preheat oven to 325°F. Insert muffin liners into the tins

In a large bowl mash bananas. Add water, oil, egg mixture and mix at low speed

Stir the spices together to mix well, then mix them with the cake mix and oatmeal.

Add the mixed dry ingredients to the wet ingredients mixture beating at low speed for 1 minute, then at high speed for 2 to 3 minutes. Do not overmix

Fold in walnuts and cranberries

Measure batter into each muffin bowl filling about 3/4 full. Do not overfill or muffins will rise and overflow out of the pan making it difficult to remove without breaking once baked.

Bake for 15 - 20 minutes or until light brown. Muffin tops will look a bit cracked.

Cool before serving or may eat them hot topped with favorite fruit spread or peanut butter for an extra kick.

Muffins freeze well if tightly sealed in a plastic bag or freezer storage container. Thaw at room temperature..

Per Serving (excluding unknown items): 139 Calories; 8g Fat (50.3% calories from fat); 2g Protein; 16g Carbohydrate; 1g Dietary Fiber; 0mg Cholesterol; 100mg Sodium. Exchanges: 0 Grain(Starch); 0 Lean Meat; 0 Fruit; 1 1/2 Fat; 1 Other Carbohydrates.

Easy Vanilla Muffins

A great any time snack. High in fiber and moderate in calories.
If using Old Fashioned oatmeal soak in water/oil/egg mixture, if using Quick Cooking add to cake mix & proceed without soaking

Yield: 24 medium
Ingredients
1 Cup Applesauce, Unsweetened
1 Cup water
1/2 Cup Vegetable Oil
1 Cup oatmeal
1 Tablespoon Vanilla, or may use another preferred spice
1 Envelope cake mix, we used Duncan Hines vanilla, white or yellow cake mix
Servings: 24

Preparation Time: 20 minutes
Start to Finish Time: 1 hour
Method

Preheat oven to 325°F. Insert muffin liners into the tins.

In a large bowl mix water, oil, egg mixture and mix at low speed. If using Old Fashioned Oatmeal add, stir to mix and soak for 30 minutes. If using Quick Cooking add with cake mix and proceed.

Add cake mix beating at low speed for 1 minute, then at high speed for 2 to 3 minutes. Do not overmix

Add flour & oatmeal mixture to wet ingredients. Stir gently until combined. Do not overmix and do not beat.

TO BAKE

Measure batter into each muffin bowl filling about 3/4 full. Do not overfill or muffins will rise and overflow out of the pan making it difficult to remove without breaking once baked.

Bake for 15 - 20 minutes or until light brown. Muffin tops will look a bit cracked.

Cool before serving or may eat them hot topped with favorite fruit spread or peanut butter for an extra kick.

Muffins freeze well if tightly sealed. Thaw at room temperature and warm in microwave or toaster oven.

Per Serving (excluding unknown items): 123 Calories; 6g Fat (46.7% calories from fat); 1g Protein; 15g Carbohydrate; 1g Dietary Fiber; 0mg Cholesterol; 100mg Sodium. Exchanges: 0 Grain(Starch); 0 Fruit; 1 1/2 Fat; 1 Other Carbohydrates.

Home-made Blueberry Muffins

1) Change it up with any berries in season
2) May use frozen or fresh berries
A great breakfast or any time snack. High in anti-inflammatory vitamins and fiber

Yield: 1 dozen

Ingredients

1 Cup Frozen Blueberries
1/3 Cup applesauce, unsweetened
1 Cup buttermilk
1 Teaspoon vanilla extract
1/2 Teaspoon baking soda
2 Teaspoons baking powder
1/2 Teaspoon salt
1 Cup oatmeal, - Quick cooking NOT instant
3/4 Cup brown sugar, - light or dark, not packed
1 Cup flour, whole-grain wheat

Servings: 12

Preparation Time: 30 minutes

Method

Preheat oven to 350°F. Insert muffin liners into the tins

In a large bowl mix frozen blueberries applesauce, buttermilk and vanilla. Stir until blended.

In a separate bowl combine flour, baking soda, baking powder, salt, cinnamon and oatmeal.

Add flour mixture to wet ingredients. Stir gently until combined. Do not overmix and do not beat.

Measure batter into each muffin bowl filling about 3/4 full. Do not overfill or muffins will rise and overflow out of the pan making it difficult to remove without breaking once baked.

Bake for 15 - 20 minutes or until light brown. Muffin tops will look a bit cracked.

Cool before serving or may eat them hot topped with favorite fruit spread or peanut butter for an extra kick.

Muffins freeze well if tightly sealed. Thaw at room temperature and warm in microwave or toaster oven.

Per Serving (excluding unknown items): 113 Calories; 1g Fat (6.7% calories from fat); 3g Protein; 24g Carbohydrate; 2g Dietary Fiber; 1mg Cholesterol; 249mg Sodium. Exchanges: 1 Grain(Starch); 0 Fruit; 0 Non-Fat Milk; 0 Fat; 1/2 Other Carbohydrates.

Jalapeño Cornbread

A spicy cornbread sure to delight your guests. Save the extras for mid-day satisfying snacks

Yield: 5 1/2 cups batter

Ingredients

1 1/2 Cups flour, whole-grain wheat
1 1/2 Cups flour, all-purpose
1 Cup cornmeal, whole-grain
2 Tablespoons baking powder
1/2 Teaspoon salt
2 Sticks unsalted butter, melted & cooled
3 Each eggs, beaten
2 Cups nonfat milk, - may use nonfat evaporated milk or buttermilk
1 Can Jalapeño Chile Peppers, drained, rinsed and finely chopped
1 Cup frozen corn kernels
Serving Ideas: 1- Bake in lined muffin tins to shorten baking time

Servings: 24

Preparation Time: 30 minutes
Start to Finish Time: 1 hour
Method

Preheat oven to 350°F

Mix dry ingredients and set aside

Mix wet ingredients and whisk to mix well

Add wet to dry ingredients including chopped jalapeños and frozen corn, mixing until all dry ingredients are wet and mixture is well mixed. Do not overmix

Let this sit at room temperature for 20 minutes then pour into prepared pan

Bake in a greased loaf pan for 45 to 55 minutes

Per Serving (excluding unknown items): 163 Calories; 9g Fat (47.2% calories from fat); 4g Protein; 18g Carbohydrate; 2g Dietary Fiber; 48mg Cholesterol; 189mg Sodium. Exchanges: 1 Grain(Starch); 0 Lean Meat; 0 Vegetable; 0 Non-Fat Milk; 1 1/2 Fat; 0 Other Carbohydrates.

Pumpkin Bread Pudding

A delicious dessert that is not too sweet. Rich enough to satisfy your sweet taste, yet amazingly low in fat.

1) Suggested toppings: crème fraiche, whipped cream, Caramel Sauce or Whipped Brandy Sauce**

** = recipes available*

Ingredients

16 cups cubed French bread, break into 1" cubes

2 cans low-fat evaporated milk, undiluted

2 cups skim milk

1 15 oz can coconut cream, canned, undiluted

1 teaspoon vanilla extract

1 1/2 cups dark brown sugar

1 cup sugar

2 tsp cinnamon

1 tsp nutmeg

1 tsp ginger

tsp salt

7 each eggs

1 15 oz canned pumpkin

2 cups Craisins, or raisins

Serving Ideas: 1-Top with Whipped Brandy Sauce

2-Serve hot or cold, plain or with your choice of toppings.

3-If you like nuts you may add 2 cups and toss to mix thoroughly at this point. Or you may wait until after the next step and sprinkle on top before baking.

Suggested Wine: A semi-sweet wine such as Rhine or Gewirstemeiner

Servings: 24

Preparation Time: 1 hour 30 minutes

Method

To make your own bread cubes use French rolls, buns or bread. Let it sit out overnight or dry in a 250°F oven for 20 - 30 minutes.

Mix all ingredients well whisking together until blended and sugars dissolved.

Pour over cubed bread tossing lightly to wet all cubes thoroughly.

If you like nuts you may add 2 cups and toss to mix thoroughly at this point. Or you may wait until after the next step and sprinkle on top before baking.

Pour into well buttered baking pans and spread evenly. Allow some of the bread crumbs to stick up so they'll toast during baking to add crunchiness. Let it sit for 20 - 30 minutes so bread cubes soak most but not all the liquid mixture

Bake in 350°F oven for 55 minutes. Do not remove when done. Turn off oven and let bread pudding sit for another 15 minutes to dry out the center.

Per Serving (excluding unknown items): 259 Calories; 5g Fat (18.4% calories from fat); 7g Protein; 47g Carbohydrate; 3g Dietary Fiber; 63mg Cholesterol; 192mg Sodium. Exchanges: 1/2 Grain(Starch); 0 Lean Meat; 1/2 Vegetable; 1/2 Fruit; 1/2 Non-Fat Milk; 1 Fat; 1 1/2 Other Carbohydrates.

Southern Style Cornbread

A fluffy Southern style cornbread. Better than a mix and just as easy

Yield: 5 1/2 cups batter

Ingredients

1 1/2 Cups flour, whole-grain wheat
1 1/2 Cups flour, all-purpose
1 Cup cornmeal, whole-grain
1 Tablespoon brown sugar
2 Tablespoons baking powder
1/2 Teaspoon salt
2 Sticks unsalted butter, cooled
3 Each eggs
2 Cups Buttermilk

Serving Ideas:

Servings: 24

Preparation Time: 30 minutes
Start to Finish Time: 1 hour

Method

Preheat oven to 350°F

Mix dry ingredients and set aside

Mix wet ingredients and whisk to mix well

Add wet to dry ingredients mixing until all dry ingredients are wet and mixture is well mixed. Do not overmix

Let this sit at room temperature for 20 minutes then pour into prepared pan

Bake for 30 to 45 minutes

Per Serving (excluding unknown items): 160 Calories; 9g Fat (49.0% calories from fat); 4g Protein; 17g Carbohydrate; 1g Dietary Fiber; 48mg Cholesterol; 200mg Sodium. Exchanges: 1 Grain(Starch); 0 Lean Meat; 0 Non-Fat Milk; 1 1/2 Fat; 0 Other Carbohydrates.

Summer Fruit Compote

A nice way to use extra fruit or fruit that is beginning to over ripen. Use with winter or summer fruits, it's just as yummy and if you make enough you'll have some left for healthy snacks all week.

Ingredients
6 Each Kiwi, Raw, peeled and cubed
1 Cup Pineapple, diced fresh, canned or frozen
3 Each oranges, peeled, seeded
2 Each Sprigs Fresh Mint, or substitute dry mint flakes
2 Inch ginger root slice, peeled and chopped
1/2 Teaspoon Rosemary, flakes or fresh minced
1/4 Cup honey
1 Dash salt
3/4 Cup orange juice
1/4 Cup Lime Juice
1 Teaspoon Lime Zest
Serving Ideas: 1-Serve hot or cold
2-Top with additional cinnamon or nutmeg before serving
3-Try adding cloves for a robust fall flavor
4-Lasts 2 weeks refrigerated at 41°F
5-Great served as ice cream topper or warm over waffles
6-Nice side dish to serve with spicy strong meats
7-In the warmer seasons substitute mangos, peaches, pineapple, apricots or plums or any other summer or tropical fruits

Servings: 16

Preparation Time: 15 minutes
Start to Finish Time: 1 hour
Method

Coarsely chop unpeeled fruit. Peel, segment and chop oranges.

Place chopped fruits in sauce pan. Add juices, spices and honey

Stir to mix well, cover and simmer for 20 to 30 minutes until fruits are cooked and tender

Taste and adjust lime if needed. Add more orange juice if a juicier compote is desired

Cool covered for half an hour, then place in a covered glass or plastic container for storage

Serve hot or cold. This fruit mix is also good to serve fresh

Per Serving (excluding unknown items): 39 Calories; trace Fat (2.2% calories from fat); trace Protein; 10g Carbohydrate; 1g Dietary Fiber; 0mg Cholesterol; 17mg Sodium. Exchanges: 0 Grain(Starch); 0 Vegetable; 1/2 Fruit; 0 Fat; 1/2 Other Carbohydrates.

Vanilla Bean Coconut Ice

A delicious coconut ice cream using only 5 ingredients. Make in the ice cream maker or in a tray. Either way you'll get a luscious desert that reminds you of a tropical island.

1) Some ice cream maker instructions have the ice cream "cure" right inside the churning bowl. Others have you transfer it to another freezer safe bowl.

2) If transferring to another bowl or container be sure to freeze it for at least 4 hours so none of the ice cream will melt.

Yield: 1 quart

Ingredients

28 fluid ounces coconut milk, 2/14 ounce cans - I prefer to use "So Good" culinary grade pure coconut milk, 2/11 oz brick packs

1 tablespoon sugar

1 tablespoon brown sugar

1/4 cup honey

1 tablespoon coconut oil, or may use a flavorless a plant oil of your choice

1/8 teaspoon salt

2 pods vanilla beans, scrape center of beans with knife for about 1/4 teaspoon total

1/2 teaspoon vanilla extract

Serving Ideas: 1 - Serve with tropical fruits such as pineapple, mango, papaya, bananas

2 - Top with cinnamon before serving and serve with a cinnamon stick and a small cinnamon cookie on the side

3 - In an ice cream cone

4 - In a float or smoothie mixed with tropical juices such as pineapple

Servings: 8

Preparation Time: 30 minutes

Start to Finish Time: 5 hours

Method

Chill coconut milk to 45°F or colder if possible

In a blender, bullet or food processor mix well all ingredients listed above. When using coconut oil add last while blending at high speed as it will harden immediately

Taste and adjust sweetness. Remember that the colder a food the less sweet it tastes. If desired you may also add a bit more vanilla extract or vanilla beans

If using the ice cream maker, pour in the bowl and follow the manufacturer instructions to churn the ice cream. Do not over churn as it will become grainy

Cover and freeze the ice cream for at least 5 hours. It should be firm but creamy.

Before serving take ice cream out for about 5 minutes. Serve in bowls or ice cream cones using a hot ice cream scoop or spoon

To heat the scoop or spoon dip in very hot water and shake water off before dipping

Although this ice cream won't last long, it will keep covered in the freezer for up to a week.

Per Serving (excluding unknown items): 299 Calories; 27g Fat (75.3% calories from fat); 2g Protein; 17g Carbohydrate;2g Dietary Fiber; 0mg Cholesterol; 50mg Sodium. Exchanges: 1/2 Fruit; 5 1/2 Fat; 1 Other Carbohydrates.

Vanilla Blueberry Sundae

A creamy sundae full of calcium, protein and antioxidants. Better than ice cream

Ingredients
1 3 3/8 Oz Package instant vanilla pudding and pie filling, may substitute sugar free pudding mix for lower calories
1 Cup 1% low-fat milk
1 1/2 Cups Yogurt, Skim Milk
2 Cups blueberries, frozen
1 Tablespoon Sugar
2 Teaspoons grated orange peel
8 Cups mint leaves, chopped fine
24 Each vanilla wafer cookies

Servings: 8

Preparation Time: 30 minutes
Start to Finish Time: 1 hour
Method

In a medium bowl place pudding mix and milk.

Beat until smooth with electric mixer - about 2 minutes.

Fold in yogurt and grated orange peel. Refrigerate covered, until thickened, about 15 minutes.

In another medium bowl combine blueberries, sugar and mint. Refrigerate covered, until ready to serve.

Layer 2 vanilla wafers in bottom of dessert bowl, 1/3 cup sauce and 1/3 cup blueberries and top with 1 vanilla wafer

Per Serving (excluding unknown items): 234 Calories; 4g Fat (15.5% calories from fat); 7g Protein; 43g Carbohydrate; 7g Dietary Fiber; 2mg Cholesterol; 307mg Sodium. Exchanges: 1 Vegetable; 1/2 Fruit; 1/2 Non-Fat Milk; 1/2 Fat; 1 ½ Other Carbohydrates.

Winter Fruit Compote

A nice way to use extra fruit or fruit that is beginning to over ripen. Use with winter or summer fruits, it's just as yummy and if you make enough you'll have some left for healthy snacks all week.

Ingredients
3 each apples, raw, unpeeled
3 each pears, raw, unpeeled
3 each oranges, peeled, seeded
2 each cinnamon stick
2 inch ginger root slice, peeled and chopped
3/4 teaspoon nutmeg
1 tablespoon brown sugar, more or less to taste
1/4 cup honey
1 dash salt
3/4 cup orange juice
4 teaspoons lemon juice, no sugar
1 teaspoon lemon zest
Serving Ideas: 1-Serve hot or cold
2-Top with additional cinnamon or nutmeg before serving
3-Try adding cloves for a robust fall flavor
4-Lasts 2 weeks refrigerated at 41°F
5-Great served as ice cream topper or warm over waffles
6-Nice side dish to serve with spicy strong meats
7-In the warmer seasons substitute mangos, peaches, pineapple, apricots or plums or any other summer or tropical fruits

Preparation Time: 15 minutes
Start to Finish Time: 1 hour
Method

Coarsely chop unpeeled fruit. Peel, segment and chop oranges.

Place chopped fruits in sauce pan. Add juices, spices, brown sugar and honey

Stir to mix well, cover and simmer for 30 to 45 minutes until fruits are cooked and tender

Taste and adjust lemon and salt if needed. Add more orange juice if a juicier compote is desired

Cool covered for half an hour, then place in a covered glass or plastic container for storage

Serve hot or cold

Servings: 16

Per Serving (excluding unknown items): 74 Calories; trace Fat (3.9% calories from fat); 1g Protein; 19g Carbohydrate; 3g Dietary Fiber; 0mg Cholesterol; 18mg Sodium. Exchanges: 0 Grain(Starch); 0 Vegetable; 1 Fruit; 0 Fat; 1/2 Other Carbohydrates.

Beverages

Banana Cantaloupe Smoothie

1) ½ lb melon = 1/2 cup AP - 1 melon yields 4 cups diced
2) 1 lb banana yields 1.5 to 3 cups
High in vitamins A & C this smoothie is a kicker start of your day

Ingredients

1/2 Cup Cantaloupe, 1/2 lb melon = 1/2 cup AP - 1 melon yields 4 cups diced
1/3 Each Sliced Banana, 1 lb banana yields 1.5 to 3 cups
1 Cup plain nonfat yogurt
1 Cup Orange Juice
1 Cup Crushed Ice

Servings: 2

Preparation Time: 10 minutes

Method

Combine all ingredients in a blender and blend until smooth.

Per Serving (excluding unknown items): 151 Calories; 1g Fat (3.8% calories from fat); 8g Protein; 30g Carbohydrate; 1g Dietary Fiber; 2mg Cholesterol; 95mg Sodium. Exchanges: 1 1/2 Fruit; 1/2 Non-Fat Milk.

Berry Pineapple Smoothie

A very satisfying beverage packed with anti-inflammatory goodness - it is recommended to buy organic or use home grown whenever possible

1) Use your favorite frozen or fresh berries

2) If using fresh berries add 1/2 cup crushed ice to chill

Ingredients	Preparation Time: 15 minutes
2 cups Almond Milk, Silk (or may substitute coconut milk or skim milk)	Method
1 teaspoon fresh ginger (1" piece grated - or may substitute 1/2 tsp ground ginger powder)	Mix all ingredients in a blender and process on high until smooth
1/2 cup pineapple chunks in juice (may use fresh, frozen or canned)	May strain if desired and process again with crushed ice to chill rapidly
1/4 each banana	
1/4 cup Frozen Blueberries	Best when icy cold
1/8 teaspoon black pepper	
1 pinch cayenne pepper	
Servings: 2	

Per Serving (excluding unknown items): 92 Calories; 3g Fat (26.1% calories from fat); 2g Protein; 16g Carbohydrate; 2g Dietary Fiber; 0mg Cholesterol; 169mg Sodium. Exchanges: 0 Grain (Starch); 0 Vegetable; 1 Fruit; 0 Fat.

Berry Breakfast Cocktail

Get your fruits and calcium in one delicious drink

1) If using fresh berries add ½ cup crushed ice to chill

Yield: 2 Cups

Ingredients

1 Cup milk, skim

1/2 Cup berries, frozen

1 Cup Orange Juice

Servings: 2

Preparation Time: 10 minutes

Method

In a blender puree all ingredients until smooth

Garnish with a mint sprig, orange wedge or more berries

Per Serving (excluding unknown items): 110 Calories; 1g Fat (4.7% calories from fat); 5g Protein; 21g Carbohydrate; 1g Dietary Fiber; 2mg Cholesterol; 65mg Sodium. Exchanges: 1 Fruit; 1/2 Non-Fat Milk.

Carrot Ginger Tonic

An anti-inflammatory refreshing drink - it is recommended to buy organic or use home grown whenever possible
1) May add more honey if a sweeter taste is preferred, or omit completely
2) May sweeten with Agave if desired

Yield: 2 Cups

Ingredients

2 Cups coconut water (not milk, just the water)
2 Tablespoons Cinnamon
1 Tablespoon fresh ginger (1" piece fresh & grated - or may substitute 1/2 tsp ground ginger powder)
2 Tablespoons lemon juice
1 Medium Grated Carrot
1/3 Each banana
1/8 Teaspoon black pepper
1 Pinch cayenne pepper
1 Teaspoon honey, may add more if a sweeter taste is preferred, or omit completely

Preparation Time: 15 minutes

Method

In a blender mix all ingredients in a blender and process on high until smooth

May strain if desired and process again with crushed ice to chill rapidly

Best when icy cold

Servings: 2

Per Serving (excluding unknown items): 112 Calories; 1g Fat (6.3% calories from fat); 3g Protein; 27g Carbohydrate; 5g Dietary Fiber; 0mg Cholesterol; 16mg Sodium. Exchanges: 1/2 Grain(Starch); 1/2 Vegetable; 1 Fruit; 0 Fat; 0 Other Carbohydrates.

Choconutty Shake

A high protein quick pick me up for mid-morning or a light lunch. A very satisfying drink for chocolate lovers

Yield: 2 cups

Ingredients

1/2 Cup Evaporated Skim Milk, undiluted
1 Cup skim milk
4 Tablespoons peanut butter
2 Tablespoons Chocolate syrup

Servings: 2

Preparation Time: 10 minutes

Method

Mix all ingredients in a blender or using an immersion stick blender

For an icy frothy drink add 1/3 cup crushed ice before blending

Per Serving (excluding unknown items): 325 Calories; 17g Fat (44.3% calories from fat); 17g Protein; 30g Carbohydrate; 2g Dietary Fiber; 5mg Cholesterol; 297mg Sodium. Exchanges: 1/2 Grain(Starch); 1 Lean Meat; 1 Non-Fat Milk; 2 1/2 Fat; 1/2 Other Carbohydrates.

Pineapple Turmeric Tonic

A dairy free anti-inflammatory nourishing smoothie - it is recommended to buy organic or use home grown whenever possible

Yield: 2 Cups

Preparation Time: 15 minutes

Ingredients

1 Cup coconut milk
1 Cup Almond Milk, Silk
1 Tablespoon fresh turmeric (2" piece grated - or may substitute 1 tsp ground turmeric powder)
1 Teaspoon fresh ginger (1" piece grated - or may substitute 1/2 tsp ground ginger powder)
1/2 Cup pineapple chunks in juice (or use fresh or frozen)
1/2 Each banana
1/8 Teaspoon black pepper
1 Pinch cayenne pepper
1/2 Teaspoon cinnamon

Method

In a blender mix all ingredients in a blender and process on high until smooth

May strain if desired and process again with crushed ice to chill rapidly

Best when icy cold

Servings: 2

Per Serving (excluding unknown items): 370 Calories; 30g Fat (69.2% calories from fat); 4g Protein; 26g Carbohydrate;5g Dietary Fiber; 0mg Cholesterol; 104mg Sodium. Exchanges: 0 Grain(Starch); 0 Vegetable; 1 1/2 Fruit; 6 Fat.

Sherbet Shake

Low in calories and high in protein. Perfect pick-me-up at any time.

Ingredients
4 Cups Skim Milk
2 Cups Sherbet
2 Cups Yogurt, Skim Milk
1 Tablespoon Vanilla
Serving Ideas: 1-Garnish with whipped topping.
2-For variety change the flavor of sherbet or use fruited yogurt

Method

Blend all ingredients in a blender or food processor until smooth

May top with fruit wedges or additional sherbet

Servings: 8

Per Serving (excluding unknown items): 149 Calories; 1g Fat (7.8% calories from fat); 8g Protein; 26g Carbohydrate; 0g Dietary Fiber; 28mg Cholesterol; 125mg Sodium. Exchanges: 1 Non-Fat Milk; 0 Fat; 1 Other Carbohydrates.

Breakfasts

Skinny Latté

A delicious treat at any time of the day - hot or cold it's just as good

Ingredients	Method
2 Cups Brewed Coffee, as strong as you like it	
1/2 Cup Evaporated Skim Milk, or use a low fat creamer of your choice	1. Add evaporated skim milk or your favorite low fat creamer, flavored or unflavored to hot coffee
Serving Ideas: 1. Top with reduced fat whipped topping	2. Add a sweetener of your choice
2. Sweeten with your choice of sugar substitute or honey	
3. Pour over crushed ice for a cold afternoon treat	
Servings: 2	

Per Serving (excluding unknown items): 55 Calories; trace Fat (2.1% calories from fat); 5g Protein; 8g Carbohydrate; 0g Dietary Fiber; 2mg Cholesterol; 78mg Sodium. Exchanges: 1/2 Non-Fat Milk.

Bacon Cheesewich

A meal in the hand the whole family will enjoy - a tasty treat

Yield: 8 Sandwiches

Ingredients

8 Each refrigerated crescent rolls, cold, separated
4 Slice Reduced Fat Monterey Jack Cheese, sliced
3/4 Cup skim milk
4 Slices bacon, cooked crisp, crumbled
8 Each eggs
1/8 Teaspoon black pepper

Servings: 8

Preparation Time: 30 minutes

Method

Heat oven to 375°F

Cook the bacon crisp, drain & crumble. Set aside.

Slightly beat eggs and mix with the milk. Add pepper to taste. No salt in needed - it is provided by bacon and cheese.

In hot grill, sauté chopped onions until soft. Add scrambled eggs mixture and crisp bacon and stir until eggs are cooked through or to 145°F

Separate crescent rolls and fill each one with 1/2 slice of cheese and 1 heaping tablespoon of scrambled eggs mixture.

Bake at 375°F until rolls puff and brown and cheese melts, about 15 minutes. Serve hot.

Per Serving (excluding unknown items): 350 Calories; 19g Fat (50.8% calories from fat); 26g Protein; 15g Carbohydrate; trace Dietary Fiber; 235mg Cholesterol; 655mg Sodium. Exchanges: 1/2 Grain(Starch); 3 Lean Meat; 0 Non-Fat Milk; 2Fat.

Breakfast Burritos

A great way to have a home-made breakfast on the go.
1) To lower sodium content use reduced sodium cheese and sausage & home-made salsa

Yield: 1 Ea.
Ingredients
1/2 Pound Sausage (may substitute low fat sausage)
1 Tablespoon onion, chopped
2 Tablespoons green bell pepper, chopped
1/2 Tablespoon ground black pepper
1 Tablespoon ground cumin
8 Each eggs, beaten
8 Each tortilla, whole wheat 96% fat free flour
2 Cups Shredded Co-jack Cheese
1 Cup salsa (mild or hot)
Servings: 8

Preparation Time: 30 minutes
Start to Finish Time: 45 minutes
Method

In a skillet brown the sausage and onions, drain fat then add the spices.

Whip the eggs and pour into hot skillet and scramble stirring from center to sides

Warm flour tortillas on a hot griddle.

Portion the scrambled egg-sausage mixture on the warmed tortilla, and sprinkle with the shredded cheese.

Fold the tortilla making a burrito. Serve with salsa.

Per Serving (excluding unknown items): 346 Calories; 19g Fat (49.6% calories from fat); 14g Protein; 30g Carbohydrate;3g Dietary Fiber; 231mg Cholesterol; 781mg Sodium. Exchanges: 0 Grain(Starch); 1 1/2 Lean Meat; 1/2 Vegetable; 2 ½ Fat.

Breakfast Stuffed Bagel

A protein-packed easy breakfast for any day of the week

Yield: 8 Servings

Ingredients

4 Each Bagels, split in half
4 Slice bacon, crisp & crumbled
4 Slices cheddar cheese, low-fat
4 Each eggs, whisked
1/2 Cup skim milk, prepared from non-fat dry milk
2 Tablespoons parsley, chopped or dry
1 Tablespoon red pepper flakes, optional

Servings: 8

Preparation Time: 20 minutes
Start to Finish Time: 40 minutes
Method

Toast split bagels lightly and lay on sheet pan cut side up.

In a bowl, beat eggs, skim milk and parsley until mixed.

Scramble until solid done but still a bit runny. Eggs will be heated again in the next step.

On each bagel, portion 1/4 cups scrambled eggs, 1 Tb crumbled bacon and 1 slice cheese. Place in oven at 350°F for 5 minutes until cheese melts and eggs finish cooking

Serve half a bagel per portion. May top with your favorite sauce

Per Serving (excluding unknown items): 281 Calories; 9g Fat (28.7% calories from fat); 23g Protein; 26g Carbohydrate; 1g Dietary Fiber; 121mg Cholesterol; 677mg Sodium. Exchanges: 1 1/2 Grain(Starch); 2 1/2 Lean Meat; 0 Vegetable; 0 Non-Fat Milk; 1/2 Fat.

Eggless Sausage-Potato Casserole

A rich protein rich breakfast casserole. A meal in one that can be prepared ahead and baked in the morning for a savory different treat. Great for an overnight crowd or a breakfast party.

Yield: 12

Ingredients

1 Pound sausage meat
1 Cup whole wheat bread, 1/2" cubes - slightly toasted or use croutons
1 Cup boiled potatoes, diced 1/2"
2 Cups low sodium cheddar cheese, shredded
2 Teaspoons mustard, yellow is OK but Poupon is better
1/4 Cup Jalapeño Pepper, Canned, drained and chopped, use more or less to taste
1 Teaspoon chili powder, more or less to taste
1/2 Cup tomato puree, reduced sodium
1 Cup skim milk
1 Tablespoon red chili flakes

Servings: 12

Preparation Time: 1 hour

Method

Cube bread and toast slightly in oven if it's fresh

Dice and boil potatoes, drain, cool slightly, toss to mix with bread crumbs

Brown sausage, breaking apart to crumble and drain

Mix mustard, tomato puree and milk, whisking to mix well

Layer bread and potatoes mixture in the bottom of a 3 - 4 inch baking pan.

Top with cooked sausage and half the shredded cheese

Mix mustard, tomato puree, skim milk, and chili powder, whisking to mix well and pour over layered ingredients. top with remaining shredded cheese

Top with remaining shredded cheese and sprinkle with red pepper flakes.

Bake at 325°F for 45 to 50 minutes or until bubbly and top browns.

Do not overcook. and be careful not to scorch cheese

Test for doneness by inserting a sharp knife in center, or take temperature to ensure it has reached 140°F

Cut in squares and serve hot

Per Serving (excluding unknown items): 306 Calories; 22g Fat (65.2% calories from fat); 12g Protein; 15g Carbohydrate;2g Dietary Fiber; 45mg Cholesterol; 462mg Sodium. Exchanges: 1 Grain(Starch); 1 1/2 Lean Meat; 0 Vegetable; 0 Non- Fat Milk; 3 1/2 Fat; 0 Other Carbohydrates.

English Muffin Breakfast Sandwich

A delicious and different breakfast packed with protein and good flavors. It's also a perfect late morning brunch.

1) Change it up using a sharp Cheddar cheese and crisp bacon slices. Sodium and fat will be higher.

Yield: 8 servings

Ingredients

8 Each English Muffin, Thomas
4 Each eggs, mixed
1/2 Cup Chopped Parsley
1 Tablespoon Skim Milk
2 Teaspoons Vegetable Oil
1/2 Cup Canadian Bacon, diced small
1/2 Cup Mozzarella Cheese, Part Skim Milk, shredded
16 Slices sliced tomatoes
1/4 Cup fresh parsley, chopped or use 2 TB dry parsley flakes

Servings: 8

Preparation Time: 30 minutes

Method

Toast split English muffins. Place one half on sheet pan.

Whip eggs and add milk, chopped parsley, diced Canadian bacon and shredded cheese

Heat oil in skillet and scramble egg mixture, stirring from center to edges to cook evenly and mix fillings

Portion scrambled eggs on bottom half of English muffin and top with sliced tomato

Place the second half of the English muffin on top of the stack, press down together

Bake at 350°F for 5 to heat and toast muffin top slightly

Each portion is 1 muffin sandwich

Per Serving (excluding unknown items): 274 Calories; 8g Fat (23.2% calories from fat); 14g Protein; 43g Carbohydrate;5g Dietary Fiber; 117mg Cholesterol; 517mg Sodium. Exchanges: 2 Grain (Starch); 1 Lean Meat; 2 1/2 Vegetable; 0 Non- Fat Milk; 1 Fat.

Fluffy French Toast

Begin your day the right way with this quick and easy protein packed breakfast

Yield: 16 Slices

Ingredients

2 Each egg
6 Each egg whites
1/3 Cup skim milk
1 Teaspoon vanilla extract
1 Teaspoon brown sugar
1/4 Teaspoon cinnamon
16 Slices wheat bread, day old or use crusty French bread
1 Teaspoon vegetable oil
1 Tablespoon butter

Servings: 8

Preparation Time: 30 minutes

Method

Beat egg whites with whisk in large bowl until frothy. Add milk, extract, brown sugar and cinnamon.

Dip each slice of bread in egg mixture.

In a skillet melt the butter, then place dipped bread to cook each side 2-3 minutes until browned.

Serve 2 slices per portion with your favorite syrup, powdered or brown sugar, or sliced fruit

Per Serving (excluding unknown items): 185 Calories; 5g Fat (25.9% calories from fat); 9g Protein; 25g Carbohydrate; 2gDietary Fiber; 57mg Cholesterol; 344mg Sodium. Exchanges: 1 1/2 Grain(Starch); 1/2 Lean Meat; 0 Non-Fat Milk; 1 Fat;0 Other Carbohydrates.

Old Fashioned Fluffy Pancakes

A light pancake for breakfast or snack

Yield: 12 Each

Ingredients

2 Cups All-purpose Flour
1 Tablespoon Baking Powder, level
1/2 Teaspoon Salt
1 Tablespoon Sugar
1 Tablespoon Vegetable Oil
1 Teaspoon Vanilla
1 Cup 2% Low-fat Milk
1 Egg
3 Tablespoons Melted Butter
Serving Ideas: 1- Serve with hot syrup & melted butter
2- Top with powdered or brown sugar
3- Top with fruits & whipped cream

Servings: 6

Method

Mix sifted flour, baking powder, salt, sugar.

Melt butter, mix with beaten egg & milk, and pour in the center of flour mixing immediately until smooth. Let sit for about 5 minutes

Heat oiled griddle on medium heat, scoop 1/4 cup batter. When top of pancake bubbles turn and let brown

Usual portion is 2 pancakes; recipe doubles well

Per Serving (excluding unknown items): 254 Calories; 9g Fat (32.9% calories from fat); 6g Protein; 37g Carbohydrate; 1g Dietary Fiber; 19mg Cholesterol; 501mg Sodium. Exchanges: 2 Grain(Starch); 0 Non-Fat Milk; 2 Fat; 0 Other Carbohydrates.

Tofu Breakfast Scramble

A delicious spicy eggless dish. No one will even suspect it's Tofu!
1) if using firm tofu simmer longer until most liquid evaporates
2) if using soft tofu simmer 2 minutes at most to avoid a dry product

Yield: 8 Servings
Ingredients
2 Pounds tofu
1/4 Cup ketchup
1/4 Teaspoon cayenne pepper
1/4 Teaspoon turmeric
1/4 Teaspoon salt
1/2 Teaspoon cumin
1 Teaspoon pepper
Servings: 8

Preparation Time: 20 minutes
Method

Pre heat skillet or grill on medium and brush generously with cooking oil

Add soft Tofu, heat slowly breaking with the spatula or spoon and simmer. Mixture will be crumbly and egg-like once done but do not overcook or use too high a temperature

Add ketchup, Cayenne pepper turmeric and cumin and stir. Turmeric will add yellow color making it look like real scrambled eggs

Per Serving (excluding unknown items): 96 Calories; 6g Fat (47.2% calories from fat); 9g Protein; 4g Carbohydrate; 2g Dietary Fiber; 0mg Cholesterol; 164mg Sodium. Exchanges: 0 Grain(Starch); 1 Lean Meat; 1/2 Fat; 0 Other Carbohydrates.

Entrées

Broiled Spicy Pork Chops

A subtly spicy pork chop to grill indoors or barbeque outdoors.

Yield: 8 Servings

Ingredients

8 Each Boneless Pork Sirloin Chops, 3/4" thick
1/2 cup red wine vinegar
1 Tablespoon vegetable oil
1 Tablespoon dry parsley flakes
2 Tablespoons Dijon-style mustard
1 Teaspoon Cumin Powder
1/4 Teaspoon Cayenne
1/2 Teaspoon Salt
1 Teaspoon Pepper

Servings: 8

Preparation Time: 25 minutes
Start to Finish Time: 1 hour
Method

In a bowl combine vinegar, oil, mustard and parsley; whisk until blended. Marinate chops for about 20 minutes.

Place pork chops in a baking pan, brush on both sides with the marinade mixture again, sprinkle salt, pepper, cumin & Cayenne on both sides before cooking.

Place marinated pork top loin chops on rack in broiler pan so surface of meat is 4 to 5 inches from heat or cook in an outdoor BBQ

Broil chops for 20 minutes turning and brushing with remaining marinade mixture when turned over then when done.

Per Serving (excluding unknown items): 150 Calories; 7g Fat (43.6% calories from fat); 19g Protein; 1g Carbohydrate; trace Dietary Fiber; 47mg Cholesterol; 220mg Sodium. Exchanges: 0 Grain (Starch); 2 1/2 Lean Meat; 0 Vegetable; 1/2Fat; 0 Other Carbohydrates.

Carnitas Tacos

Shredded or chopped pork, beef or turkey with beans and cheese served in a warm soft tortilla. Great way to use leftover meat

Yield: 8 Tacos

Ingredients

2 Cups Cooked Pork, may use ground beef or turkey
1 Cup Black Beans, rinsed and drained
1 Tablespoon Chile, powder
1/2 Cup chopped onion
1 Clove garlic, crushed
1 Tablespoon diced jalapeño pepper, hot or mild your choice
8 Each corn tortillas, warmed
1/2 Cup shredded lettuce
1/2 Cup diced tomatoes
1 Cup cheddar cheese, low-fat
2 Cups Salsa, as desired

Servings: 8

Preparation Time: 25 minutes

Method

In nonstick skillet, sauté onion and garlic over medium heat for 10 or 15 minutes, until soft and translucent.

Add cooked pork; toss lightly. Heat thoroughly to 145°F. Stir in jalapeño pepper. In each warm tortilla, measure 1/3 cup meat mixture, a portion of the lettuce, tomatoes, 1 heaping tablespoon cheese and top with salsa.

In each warm tortilla, measure 1/3 cup meat mixture, a portion of the lettuce, tomatoes, 1 heaping tablespoon cheese and top with salsa.

Per Serving (excluding unknown items): 320 Calories; 14g Fat (39.3% calories from fat); 20g Protein; 29g Carbohydrate;5g Dietary Fiber; 44mg Cholesterol; 161mg Sodium. Exchanges: 2 Grain (Starch); 2 Lean Meat; 1/2 Vegetable; 1 1/2 Fat.

Chile Verde

My own version of the New Mexico classic - amazingly low in calories

Yield: 8 Cups

Preparation Time: 25 minutes

Ingredients

1 1/2 Pounds boneless pork butt (shoulder)
1 Tablespoon vegetable oil
1/4 Cup chopped onion
3 Cloves garlic, minced
1 Tablespoon ground oregano
1 Tablespoon ground cumin
1 Teaspoon Salt
1 Teaspoon Pepper
1/2 Cup diced green chiles (New Mexico green chiles)
3 Cups Reduced Sodium Chicken Broth
1 Tablespoon hot pepper sauce (Tabasco)
1/2 Cup fresh cilantro, chopped

Servings: 8

Method

Dice pork butt or shoulder, dust with flour & season with black pepper

Heat oil in stock pot over medium-high heat; add pork cubes and brown evenly on all sides. Add onions and garlic to pan; cook and stir until onions are tender, about 10 minutes.

Stir in remaining ingredients and bring all to a boil. Lower heat to a simmer, cover and simmer until pork is very tender and liquid is slightly thickened.

Serve immediately over hot cooked rice, if desired. Garnish with fresh cilantro sprigs.

Per Serving (excluding unknown items): 189 Calories; 8g Fat (41.9% calories from fat); 24g Protein; 3g Carbohydrate; 1g Dietary Fiber; 68mg Cholesterol; 578mg Sodium. Exchanges: 0 Grain(Starch); 3 Lean Meat; 1/2 Vegetable; 1/2 Fat; 0 Other Carbohydrates.

Creamy Pesto Pasta

An amazingly nutritious version of pesto pasta - you won't believe how low in fat and sodium it is when you taste it.

Yield: 8 Servings

Ingredients

1 pound Whole Wheat Spaghetti
2 Cups fresh spinach, stems removed
2 Cups basil leaves
4 Each Garlic Cloves, crushed or chopped
1/4 Cup olive oil
1 Cup Half and Half
1 Teaspoon Pepper
1 Cup mozzarella cheese, part skim milk, shredded
1/2 Cup Parmesan, grated

Servings: 8

Preparation Time: 20 minutes

Method

Cook pasta al dente, drain and keep warm

Combine spinach and basil in a food processor bowl and chop fine

In a saucepan sauté garlic in olive oil at low heat to avoid scorching. When you smell the cooked garlic aroma add milk, chopped spinach and basil

Simmer for 10 minutes stirring constantly to avoid scorching or sticking

Add cooked pasta and toss to mix. Turn off heat.

Immediately add grated mozzarella & Parmesan cheeses. Toss to mix well

Per Serving (excluding unknown items): 342 Calories; 13g Fat (34.0% calories from fat); 13g Protein; 45g Carbohydrate;5g Dietary Fiber; 19mg Cholesterol; 98mg Sodium. Exchanges: 3 Grain(Starch); 1/2 Lean Meat; 0 Vegetable; 0 Non-Fat Milk; 2 1/2 Fat.

Creamy Skinny Enchiladas

Mexican food without guilt! And so easy to make!

Yield: 16 Each

Ingredients

16 Each corn tortillas
2 Teaspoons vegetable oil
1 Can Green Enchilada Sauce, choose your heat level
1 Can low sodium tomatoes, canned, diced or chopped
1/2 Can cream of chicken soup, try using reduced fat such as a 90% low fat soup
1/2 Can skim milk
2 Cups Diced Chicken
1 Cup black beans, drain and rinse canned or may cook dry beans use leftover beans
1 Cup cheddar cheese, low sodium, may substitute any preferred white, white and yellow or Mexican style cheese

Servings: 8

Preparation Time: 30 minutes
Start to Finish Time: 1 hour

Method

Lightly oil tortillas and heat to make them easier to roll without breaking.

Place tortilla on flat surface or shallow dish, spread enchilada sauce to coat evenly then add fillings in the center of each tortilla. Do not overfill so tortilla will fold

Fold tortilla by bringing each end towards the middle and overlapping. Carefully turn enchilada over and place seam down in baking dish.

If you prefer tortillas may place in overlapping layers, filling spread on top, then top with the second tortilla.

Mix remaining enchilada sauce with an equal part of tomato sauce and pour over enchiladas. Top with shredded cheese

Cover lightly with foil and bake at 350°F up to 30 minutes or until heated through and cheese melted.

Per Serving (excluding unknown items): 419 Calories; 18g Fat (37.6% calories from fat); 23g Protein; 43g Carbohydrate;7g Dietary Fiber; 62mg Cholesterol; 239mg Sodium. Exchanges: 2 1/2 Grain(Starch); 2 1/2 Lean Meat; 1/2 Vegetable; 0 Non-Fat Milk; 2 Fat.

Crispy Oven Fried Fish

Better than the ubiquitous frozen breaded fish and a lot more nutritious.

NOTE: to avoid confusion during this multi-step preparation salt and pepper have been added twice in the recipe, once for seasoning the fish the other for seasoning the egg-milk mixture

Yield: 8 Servings

Ingredients

1 Pound Cod Fillets, thawed
3/4 Cup Flour, All-purpose
1/8 Teaspoon Salt, to sprinkle on raw fish filets
1/8 Teaspoon Pepper, to sprinkle on raw fish filets
2 Each Eggs
1 Tablespoon Milk
1/4 Teaspoon Salt, to season egg-milk mixture
1/4 Teaspoon Pepper, to season egg-milk mixture
2 Cups cornflakes, crushed
4 Tablespoons Parmesan cheese, grated
1/4 Teaspoon cayenne pepper, to season cornflakes coating
1/2 Cup Tartar Sauce

Serving Ideas:

Servings: 8

Preparation Time: 1 hour

Method

Position the seasoned flour, egg-milk mixture and cornflakes-Parmesan mixture next to each other in the order given below (from left to right or right to left depending on your preference)

- Place flour in a wide bowl

- Whisk together egg, salt, pepper and milk in a second pan.

- Mix cornflakes, Parmesan and cayenne in a 2" pan.

Pat fish dry and dredge in flour on both sides

Dip dredged fish in egg-milk mixture to coat both sides, and then coat with cornflake mixture making sure all sides are covered

Place on a baking sheet that has been lightly sprayed with non-stick cooking spray. Bake at 450ºF, 10 - 15 minutes or until fish flakes when tested with a fork and coating is crunchy

Serve with Tartar Sauce

Per Serving (excluding unknown items): 221 Calories; 11g Fat (43.5% calories from fat); 15g Protein; 16g Carbohydrate; 1g Dietary Fiber; 89mg Cholesterol; 369mg Sodium. Exchanges: 1 Grain(Starch); 1 1/2 Lean Meat; 0 Fruit; 0 Non-Fat Milk; 1 1/2 Fat.

Crunchy Turkey Salad

Spicy crunchy turkey salad - high in fiber and a powerful protein pack

Yield: 8 Servings

Ingredients

1 Cup Lentils, dry, pulsed 3 times in the food processor
1 Pound cooked turkey, diced
2 Teaspoons dry parsley flakes, chopped
1 Tablespoon Red Onion, chopped fine
1/2 Cup red pepper, chopped
1/2 Cup Diced Celery
1/2 Cup light mayonnaise
1 Tablespoon Dijon Mustard
1 Cup Spinach Leaves
1 Cup Cooked Barley

Servings: 8

Preparation Time: 1 hour 20 minutes

Method

Wash lentils and pick clean. Spread on paper towel to dry while salad ingredients are mixed

Mix first next 9 ingredients in bowl and toss to coat meat and vegetables well.

Add cracked dry lentils and toss to mix well.

Cover and refrigerate for an hour before servings to blend flavors

Per Serving (excluding unknown items): 254 Calories; 8g Fat (26.6% calories from fat); 24g Protein; 23g Carbohydrate;9g Dietary Fiber; 47mg Cholesterol; 147mg Sodium. Exchanges: 1 1/2 Grain(Starch); 3 Lean Meat; 0 Vegetable; 1/2 Fat;0 Other Carbohydrates.

Cuban Style Sandwich

A nostalgic reminder of walkup sandwich bars in Cuba - if you're really hip you'll call these Cubanos and eat it with a cup of strong sweet coffee

Yield: 8 Servings

Preparation Time: 45 minutes

Ingredients

8 Each sandwich roll, 6" (French, Italian or large hotdog bun)
8 Each Ham Slices, 1 oz slices
8 Each Turkey Breast Slices, 1 oz slices
8 Each Swiss cheese, low-fat, 1 oz slices
2 Tablespoons Olive Oil
1 Tablespoon Ground Oregano

Servings: 8

Method

Spread insides of split roll with the olive oil oregano mixture.

Portion meats & cheese slices and thinly sliced pickles on rolls then cover with bun top half

Place rolls on a lightly oiled heated flat skillet or grill .

Grill for about 15 minutes pressing down lightly with spatula to flatten the bread.

Or grill in a sandwich or Panini grill until heated through but the bread is still soft

Garnish with dill pickles, olives and cherry tomatoes for a fun meal

Per Serving (excluding unknown items): 372 Calories; 14g Fat (34.8% calories from fat); 43g Protein; 17g Carbohydrate;1g Dietary Fiber; 59mg Cholesterol; 1018mg Sodium. Exchanges: 1 Grain(Starch); 5 1/2 Lean Meat; 1 1/2 Fat.

Fish Tostada

Grilled fish on crispy corn tortillas with shredded cabbage, corn & sweet lime salsa

Yield: 8 Servings

Ingredients

1 Pound fish fillets (may use another seafood or cooked fish if desired)
2 Cups black beans, cooked, drained
1 Cup frozen corn, thawed not cooked
1 Tablespoon Vegetable Oil
1/2 Cup Chopped Onion, diced fine
1/4 Cup Reduced Sodium Chicken Broth
8 Each Corn Tortilla, warmed or fried crisp, your preference
2 Cups Shredded Cabbage
1 Cup Salsa Verde
1/2 Cup Lime Juice, unsweetened
Serving Ideas: 1- This also makes a great taco
2- May also hack this recipe and use any other type of meat you prefer
3- Try it with tofu for a vegan delight

Servings: 8

Preparation Time: 45 minutes

Method

Season, grill or bake the fish filets

When ready to use, flake fish filets, then proceed with tostada filling recipe

In skillet or grill heat oil, sauté onion over medium heat for 10 to 15 minutes or until soft and translucent.

Add drained beans and corn and stir to heat.

Add flaked fish and broth and heat slowly, stirring to spread heat, to 145°F. Do not overheat or allow to dry.

Keep hot while assembling tostadas but do not overheat or allow to dry.

Mix salsa verde and lime juice and reserve until serving time

Place the hot tortillas on plates and top with the fish-vegetable mixture on top of each tortilla.

Top with 1/2 cup shredded cabbage and top with 1 Tb lime-chile salsa mixture

Per Serving (excluding unknown items): 215 Calories; 3g Fat (13.0% calories from fat); 16g Protein; 31g Carbohydrate; 6g Dietary Fiber; 24mg Cholesterol; 184mg Sodium. Exchanges: 1 1/2 Grain(Starch); 1 1/2 Lean Meat; 1/2 Vegetable; 0 Fruit; 1/2 Fat.

Grilled Cheese Italiano

The flavors of Italy in a simple, hearty grilled cheese sandwich. A savory switch to a traditional stand-by.

Ingredients

16 Slices Italian bread, sliced 1" thick
1 Pound mozzarella cheese, part skim milk, sliced
1 Tablespoon Romano cheese, grated
1 Tablespoon low calorie Italian salad dressing, emulsified
3 Cups shredded carrots
1 Cup basil leaves, chopped
2 Each Garlic Cloves, crushed or chopped
1/2 Cup black olives, chopped or sliced
4 Each Roma Tomato, sliced thin
16 Each romaine lettuce leaves
1 Tablespoon Olive Oil, to coat skillet when grilling

Servings: 8

Preparation Time: 45 minutes

Method

Mince or crush garlic and mix with olive oil. A mortar and pestle make this quick and easy

Brush oil garlic mixture to one side of each of the 2 bread slices

Layer mozzarella cheese slices, shredded carrots, sliced tomatoes and chopped olives on one slice and top with second slice.

Press bread down lightly, being careful not to tear it. When ready to grill pick up carefully so they don't fall apart.

To grill, brush a medium hot skillet with olive oil and toast the sandwiches on both sides until cheese is melted.

Per Serving (excluding unknown items): 334 Calories; 14g Fat (38.6% calories from fat); 21g Protein; 31g Carbohydrate;4g Dietary Fiber; 32mg Cholesterol; 655mg Sodium. Exchanges: 1 1/2 Grain(Starch); 2 Lean Meat; 1 1/2 Vegetable; 0 Fruit; 1 1/2 Fat; 0 Other Carbohydrates.

Hearty Sausage Pizza

A quick and easy pizza, but oh! so delicious don't be surprised if you run out

Yield: 2 Pizzas

Ingredients

2 Each Pizza Dough, 9" to 10"

2 Tablespoons olive oil

2 Tablespoons Italian Seasoning, or sodium free herbs

1 Pound mozzarella cheese, part skim milk, shredded

1 Cup Ricotta Cheese

1/2 Pound bulk low fat Italian sausage, if you like it hot try the spicy

1/2 Cup spicy pizza sauce, or may use enchilada sauce

1/2 Cup marinara sauce, or may use your favorite pasta sauce

Servings: 8

Preparation Time: 20 minutes

Start to Finish Time: 1 hour

Method

Pre-heat oven to 450°F

Roll out pizza crust and place on 2 lightly oiled pizza pans or sheet pan

Brown the sausage and pour out grease. Add the sauces and mix well.

Brush tops of pizza crust lightly with oil, sprinkle with sodium free Italian seasoning herbs

Evenly divide all ingredients between both pans layering first the Ricotta, then the grated mozzarella and then the sausage-sauce mixture

Bake at 450°F for 30 minutes until cheese is melted and crust the desired color

Sprinkle with grated Parmesan cheese and red hot pepper flakes if desired

Per Serving (excluding unknown items): 556 Calories; 29g Fat (47.4% calories from fat); 29g Protein; 44g Carbohydrate;1g Dietary Fiber; 68mg Cholesterol; 698mg Sodium. Exchanges: 2 1/2 Grain(Starch); 3 Lean Meat; 1/2 Vegetable; 4 Fat.

Jiffy Traditional Enchiladas

On a very busy day there's nothing better than a quick and easy hot meal

Yield: 8 Servings

Ingredients

1 Pound ground turkey

1/2 Cup onion, chopped

1/3 Cup diced green chiles, mild or hot - pick your favorite heat level

1 Cup enchilada sauce, canned

1 Cup cream of mushroom soup, undiluted

1/2 Pound Grated Cheddar Cheese

16 Each corn tortillas

Serving Ideas: 1- May use ground or shredded beef, pork, chicken or fish

Servings: 8

Preparation Time: 20 minutes

Start to Finish Time: 45 minutes

Method

Brown ground meat and chopped onion, pour off grease.

Mix 1/2 cup of cream of mushroom soup and 1/2 cup enchilada sauce and set aside for later use.

Add remaining ingredients to the cooked ground turkey but not cheese and reserved sauce, and simmer for 60 minutes until flavors blend well

Spray a 2" baking pan lightly with food release to prevent sticking and spread the reserved 1 cup of sauce and soup mixture evenly on the bottom to coat pan

Lay half the tortillas on the bottom of pan evenly, overlapping slightly to fit inside the pan

Portion the sauce over the tortillas and cover with the remaining half of the tortillas.

Sprinkle the cheese evenly over the top. Bake in hot oven at 350°F for 15 minutes until cheese melts. Do not overheat or cheese and tortillas will harden

To portion, cut into 8 squares and serve hot.

Garnish with additional sauce, avocado, guacamole or sour cream

Per Serving (excluding unknown items): 287 Calories; 13g Fat (38.9% calories from fat); 15g Protein; 30g Carbohydrate;3g Dietary Fiber; 61mg Cholesterol; 518mg Sodium. Exchanges: 1 1/2 Grain(Starch); 1 1/2 Lean Meat; 1/2 Vegetable; 11/2 Fat.

Magic Marinated Chicken

A little bit pungent, a little bit sweet and very savory chicken - 3 robust flavors in one

Yield: 8 each

Ingredients

2 Tablespoons Paprika
1 Teaspoon Chili Powder
1 Teaspoon black pepper
2 Tablespoons Brown Sugar
1 Tablespoon Garlic Powder
1/4 Cup Balsamic Vinegar
1/4 Tablespoon Olive Oil
2 Tablespoons Low Sodium Soy Sauce
1 Teaspoon Worcestershire Sauce
1 Tablespoon Lemon Juice
1 Tablespoon Dijon Mustard
1 Tablespoon Flour, All-purpose
8 Each Skinless Chicken Breast Halves, bone-in skin removed

Servings: 8

Preparation Time: 3 hours 30 minutes

Method

In a large bowl mix the marinade ingredients and (the first 12 listed) whisk to mix well

Place cold chicken breasts in a 2" or deeper glass baking dish and pour the marinade coating it well

Cover and refrigerate for up to 4 hours

Remove chicken from the marinade placing on a rack to drain, then dredge chicken pieces in the flour

Layer chicken in a foil lined 1" baking sheet and bake in a 350° oven for 45-60 minutes or until internal temperature reaches 170°F. Turn for even browning.

Per Serving (excluding unknown items): 162 Calories; 2g Fat (12.9% calories from fat); 28g Protein; 6g Carbohydrate; 1g Dietary Fiber; 68mg Cholesterol; 261mg Sodium. Exchanges: 0 Grain(Starch); 4 Lean Meat; 0 Vegetable; 0 Fruit; 0 Fat;0 Other Carbohydrates.

Meatloaf Muffin Cups

Pre-portioned meatloaf muffins. Great for a meal and even better for a high protein snack. Make in advance and freeze for later.

Yield: 24 each

Ingredients

2 pounds lean ground beef, may substitute turkey or pork
1/2 cup diced tomatoes, crushed or mashed
1 cup vegetable juice, low sodium or low sodium spicy version
1 cup grated carrots
1 1/4 cups oatmeal, old fashioned
1/2 cup green onion, finely chopped
2 each eggs, slightly beaten
2 tablespoons Worcestershire sauce
1 tablespoon soy sauce, low sodium
2 teaspoons dried thyme leaves
1 tablespoon garlic powder
1/2 teaspoon pepper

Servings: 24

Preparation Time: 30 minutes
Start to Finish Time: 1 hour

Method

Heat oven to 350ºF. In large bowl, combine ground beef, vegetable juice, green onion, eggs, Worcestershire & soy sauces, thyme, garlic powder, pepper and dry mustard. Toss lightly to mix thoroughly.

Grease inside of up cake pans with oil or pan release. Spoon meat mixture in muffin pans filling them 3/4 full.

Bake in 350ºF oven 20 minutes or until no longer pink and juices run clear.

Top with brown gravy or your favorite sauce

1 portion = 2 muffins

Per Serving (excluding unknown items): 131 Calories; 9g Fat (59.6% calories from fat); 8g Protein; 5g Carbohydrate; 1g Dietary Fiber; 46mg Cholesterol; 109mg Sodium. Exchanges: 0 Grain(Starch); 1 Lean Meat; 1/2 Vegetable; 1 Fat; 0 Other Carbohydrates.

Mediterranean Rollup

1) Hummus recipe available
Vegan with option to add cheese or meat

Yield: 8 Each

Ingredients

8 each tortillas, whole wheat 96% fat free flour, 8" size rolls up best. May also use Lavash or corn tortillas
1 cup hummus, home-made or purchased
1 cup romaine lettuce leaves, chopped
2 cups Canned Black Beans, drained & rinsed
4 each tomatoes, red ripe, chopped
1 cup kale, or red tip romaine lettuce
2 tablespoons black olives, chopped
4 tablespoons low calorie Italian salad dressing, emulsified

Servings: 8

Preparation Time: 45 minutes

Method

Toss cooked black beans with 1 tablespoon dressing and coarsely mash

Lay out tortillas on a flat surface and spread each with hummus then spread the mashed black beans on top

Toss the chopped lettuce, kale, tomatoes and black olives with remaining 1 tablespoon dressing

Roll starting from the edge of a long side, roll it up. Cut diagonally in half.

To store wrap in plastic wrap, seal the ends and refrigerate at 41°F until serving time.

Per Serving (excluding unknown items): 278 Calories; 7g Fat (22.9% calories from fat); 11g Protein; 44g Carbohydrate; 9g Dietary Fiber; trace Cholesterol; 787mg Sodium. Exchanges: 1 Grain(Starch); 1/2 Lean Meat; 1 Vegetable; 0 Fruit; 1/2 Fat; 0 Other Carbohydrates.

Rustic Summer Sandwich

An open face assembled sandwich. A fun project for children to make their own using their favorite fillings

Yield: 1 Each

Ingredients

6 slices sourdough bread
3 Sliced Zucchini, or other summer squash
3 Sliced Tomatoes
3/4 Cup avocado, mashed
1 1/2 cloves garlic, crushed
2 Tablespoons parmesan cheese, grated
1 Tablespoon lime juice, freshly squeezed
Serving Ideas: Garnish with chopped green or black olives, Italian parsley, green onion tops or pimento slices

Servings: 6

Method

Toast one side of thick slice of freshly baked sour dough whole wheat bread. Rub with peeled garlic clove

Crush the remaining garlic cloves and mix with enough mashed avocado to make 3/4 cups. Spread 2 TB avocado. Squeeze a few drops of fresh lemon or lime

Spread toasted side of bread with 2 tablespoons avocado & top with a few drops of lime juice to keep from browning

Top with very thin slices of fresh zucchini or other summer squash and thick slices of tomato

Sprinkle with pinch of Kosher or sea salt & generous grinder of pepper

Top with Parmesan cheese to taste, either grated or ribboned

If desired both sides of the bread can be toasted, but this makes it harder to eat as it's crunchier and crumbles

After sandwich is assembled the open face sandwich can be grilled to brown the bottom and heat the filling slightly

Per Serving (excluding unknown items): 134 Calories; 4g Fat (27.9% calories from fat); 5g Protein; 21g Carbohydrate; 3g Dietary Fiber; 1mg Cholesterol; 194mg Sodium. Exchanges: 1 Grain (Starch); 0 Lean Meat; 1 Vegetable; 0 Fruit; 1/2 Fat.

Tarragon Chicken Breasts

Take a flavor trip through the Mediterranean with this delicious dish

Yield: 8 Servings

Ingredients

1 Pound Boneless Skinless Chicken Breast, 8 pieces
1 1/2 Cups bread crumbs
1 Cup Flour
1/2 Cup Buttermilk
1 Each Egg
1/4 Cup Dijon Mustard
1 Tablespoon Garlic Powder, crushed
2 Tablespoons minced flat-leaf parsley
2 Tablespoons minced fresh tarragon
1 Teaspoon freshly ground pepper
2 Cups Flour
1/2 Cup olive oil

Servings: 8

Preparation Time: 1 hour 30 minutes

Method

Preheat oven to 350°F

Line up 3 shallow bowls: 1: flour, 2: bread crumbs with herbs, garlic powder, parsley, tarragon & pepper, 3: egg, buttermilk, mustard

Dredge each chicken breast in flour; dip in egg and then bread crumb mixture, covering completely and patting so crumbs adhere.

Line a sheet pan with foil with the shiny side up. Lightly brush foil with olive oil and place breaded chicken breasts with space between them to allow browning

Bake at 350°F for 30 - 40 minutes, testing internal temperature to ensure meat is cooked through.

Per Serving (excluding unknown items): 458 Calories; 17g Fat (33.6% calories from fat); 22g Protein; 53g Carbohydrate;2g Dietary Fiber; 60mg Cholesterol; 332mg Sodium. Exchanges: 3 1/2 Grain(Starch); 2 Lean Meat; 0 Vegetable; 0 Non- Fat Milk; 3 Fat; 0 Other Carbohydrates.

Turkey Caesar Wrap

Better than a sandwich and not as messy. Wraps take minutes to make & are the latest rage.

Yield: 8 Wraps

Ingredients

1 Cup Caesar Salad Dressing, homogenized
8 Each 10-inch Fat-free Flour Tortilla
2 Cups Romaine Lettuce, chopped
1 Cup Kale, chopped
1 Cup Red Bell Pepper, chopped
2 Cups cooked turkey, pulled or diced
1/2 Cup Parmesan cheese

Servings: 8

Preparation Time: 1 hour 45 minutes

Method

Warm tortillas to make them easier to roll without breaking

Spread a generous 2 to 3 tablespoons Caesar dressing over entire surface of each flour tortilla.

Toss all ingredients together with dressing to coat with dressing to mix well

Divide evenly on the center of each tortilla, tuck in a long end to overlap with and seal the filling - like making a burrito

Roll up each sandwich tightly like a jelly roll; lay down on seam side until done rolling.

Wrap each roll-up with plastic wrap tightly enough to hold them together. Refrigerate 1 hour.

Cut each wrap diagonally before serving. 1 portion = 2 halves

May serve with additional dressing on the side

Per Serving (excluding unknown items): 357 Calories; 8g Fat (21.9% calories from fat); 19g Protein; 49g Carbohydrate;3g Dietary Fiber; 31mg Cholesterol; 767mg Sodium. Exchanges: 2 1/2 Grain(Starch); 1 1/2 Lean Meat; 1/2 Vegetable; 1Fat; 1/2 Other Carbohydrates.

Vegetable Quesadillas

Change the pace for lunch. Make a hot finger-food much tastier than a sandwich

Yield: 8 Each

Ingredients

8 Each Tortilla, Whole Wheat 96% Fat Free Flour
1 Tablespoon Vegetable Oil, divided to use half at a time during cooking
1/4 Cup Red Onion, chopped
3/4 Cup Shredded Carrot
3/4 Cup Shredded Zucchini
3/4 Cup Chopped Tomatoes
1/2 Cup Tomato Puree
1/4 Cup Canned Jalapeño Peppers, drained and chopped
2 Cups Cheddar Cheese, Low-fat Serving Ideas: 1) For authentic Mexican flavor season with Mexican Seasoning (recipe available) and use Cotija or another Mexican cheese

Servings: 8

Preparation Time: 45 minutes

Method

Heat half the oil in a skillet or sauce pan. Add onions and carrot and cook over low heat 3 minutes or until onion is soft but not brown. Stir in tomatoes and jalapenos - cook until just heated through.

Heat tortillas to make them easier to fold without splitting and spread them on a warm baking sheet

Spread the seasoned tomatoes mixture in the first step on each tortilla

Evenly divide the shredded vegetables on one half of each tortilla. If any seasoned tomato sauce is left spoon on top of the fillings. Fold the second half of the tortilla on top and press down to flatten.

Heat the remaining oil in a large flat non-stick skillet or hot grill. Cook one or two quesadillas at a time about 30 seconds per side until lightly browned on both sides, cheese melts and filling is heated

One portion is one folded quesadilla

Per Serving (excluding unknown items): 223 Calories; 6g Fat (25.1% calories from fat); 12g Protein; 31g Carbohydrate;3g Dietary Fiber; 6mg Cholesterol; 674mg Sodium. Exchanges: 1 Lean Meat; 1 Vegetable; 1/2 Fat.

Wild West Burgers

When you want a great new taste in your burgers try this quick recipe

Ingredients

2 Pounds Ground Turkey, may substitute 4 - 4 oz lean turkey patties
1 Tablespoon Mexican Seasoning, recipe available
1/2 Cup Shredded Cheddar Cheese
8 Each Hamburger Bun, Mixed Grain
1 Cup Salsa
Serving Ideas: 1) May use lean beef or beef patties
2) Try it with a skinless boneless chicken breast seasoned with Mexican Seasoning (recipe available)

Servings: 8

Preparation Time: 30 minutes

Method

In bowl, combine meat and Mexican seasonings mix and mix well. Add shredded cheese and toss to mix again

Form 8 patties (each patty should weigh about 5 ounces). Before cooking top each with 1 tablespoon salsa, reserving the remainder to use in the sandwich

Grill until juices run clear or 165°F internal temperature

Per Serving (excluding unknown items): 354 Calories; 15g Fat (38.5% calories from fat); 31g Protein; 24g Carbohydrate;2g Dietary Fiber; 89mg Cholesterol; 554mg Sodium. Exchanges: 1 1/2 Grain(Starch); 4 Lean Meat; 1/2 Vegetable; 1 Fat.

Zany Beef and Mushroom Stew

Robust flavors are easy to achieve with this simple recipe - cooked in the oven on a cold winter day On a hot day use your InstantPot for an easy fool proof meal

Yield: 8 Cups

Preparation Time: 4 hours

Ingredients

1 1/2 Pounds beef stew meat, remove fat & gristle
4 Cups Mushrooms, stems removed
1 Pound new potatoes, cut in half
1/2 Pound carrot slices, slice or cut in 1" chunks
3 Cups canned tomatoes, with juice
2 Cups Chopped Green Bell Pepper, or try using 1/2 hoot & 1/2 mild peppers
1 Tablespoon onion powder
1 Tablespoon garlic powder
2 Teaspoons pepper, 1/2 tsp each or to taste
2 Each bay leaf, remove before serving
2 Cups fresh parsley, or use 1/4 cup dry parsley flakes
1 Teaspoon Rosemary, powder
2 Teaspoons thyme, powder
2 Cups Reduced Sodium Chicken Broth
1 Cup Red Wine, use a good quality Cabernet
2 2/3 Tablespoons all-purpose flour
2/3 Cup water

Servings: 8

Method

Heat oven to 375°F. In 4-quart ovenproof bean pot or casserole, place all ingredients except water, wine, flour and vegetables

Cook in oven for 1 1/2 to 2 hours until meat is tender

While meat cooks, prepare remaining ingredients: cutting the unpeeled potatoes in half, slice carrots and peppers in 1" pieces

In small bowl mix cold water and flour and temper with an equal amount of hot broth from the meat

Gradually stir tempered thickening mixture into beef mixture

Cover and simmer again for at least 1/2 hour or until meat and vegetables are tender

Add wine, stir and adjust seasonings. If the gravy is too thin remove cover to reduce liquid, if too thick add wine or broth

Per Serving (excluding unknown items): 283 Calories; 8g Fat (26.8% calories from fat); 23g Protein; 26g Carbohydrate;5g Dietary Fiber; 47mg Cholesterol; 363mg Sodium. Exchanges: 1 Grain (Starch); 2 1/2 Lean Meat; 2 Vegetable; 0 Fat.

Salads
& Sides

Barley Corn Pilaf

A spicy high fiber side dish; salad, vegetable and starch all in one - an amazing picnic dish since it's good either hot, cold or at room temperature

Yield: 8 Cups

Ingredients

2 Tablespoons Extra virgin olive oil
1/4 Cup chopped onions, may substitute 1 teaspoon onion powder
1/2 Cup chopped parsley, may substitute 1 tablespoon dry parsley flakes
1 Cup pearl barley
1/2 Teaspoon Salt, in barley water
3/4 Cup red peppers, chopped
2 cups Reduced Sodium Chicken Broth, homemade is best but may use canned or brick packed
1 Cup frozen corn kernels
1 Cup frozen peas
2 Tablespoons fresh ginger root, peeled and chopped
1 Teaspoon ground turmeric
1 Teaspoon curry powder
1 Teaspoon black pepper
2 Teaspoons red pepper flakes
2 Tablespoons Italian Salad Dressing

Servings: 8

Preparation Time: 1 hour 30 minutes

Method

In a 2 quart sauce pan sauté onions in olive oil until clear

Add barley, stir to mix and coat with the oil.

Add chicken broth, pepper, turmeric and curry. Stir to dissolve spices and mix well.

Cook at medium heat (small bubbles) until barley is tender.

Add frozen corn and peas, 2 teaspoons red pepper flakes and remaining. Stir from bottom up to mix well

Remove from heat, cover and let stand until all liquid is absorbed and vegetables are tender but still crunchy

If desired adjust seasoning and add more broth for a juicier dish

Garnish with chopped fresh parsley and fresh red pepper

Serve steaming hot or cold on a lettuce bed

Per Serving (excluding unknown items): 180 Calories; 6g Fat (27.9% calories from fat); 5g Protein; 29g Carbohydrate; 6g Dietary Fiber; 0mg Cholesterol; 323mg Sodium. Exchanges: 2 Grain (Starch); 1/2 Vegetable; 0 Fruit; 1 Fat.

Cauliflower Chopped Salad

A refreshing summer or winter salad. It can be made into a side dish, salad or complete meal.

Yield: 12 Cups

Ingredients

2 Pounds Cauliflower, fresh, wash, core
1 Cup cucumber, chopped
6 Each tomatoes, quartered
1 Bunch flat leaf parsley, chopped
1/4 Cup cilantro, chopped
1 Tablespoon chopped basil
2 Cloves garlic, minced fine
1 Tablespoon Lemon Juice, squeeze & zest
1 Teaspoon Lemon Zest
1/3 Cup extra virgin olive oil
1 Teaspoon kosher salt
1 Teaspoon pepper, black or white

Serving Ideas: 1- For a complete meal add your choice of 1-1/2 pounds of diced meats, fish or tofu as desired and serve 1-1/2 cups per portions

Servings: 12

Preparation Time: 30 minutes
Start to Finish Time: 30 minutes

Method

Cut cauliflower in half, core, wash and drain

Cut each half into florets small enough to fit through food processor feeder tube

Process in batches until small. Do not over process - stop once the batch looks uniform. Remove each batch to a large mixing or serving bowl

Stir in the cucumbers, tomatoes & chopped herbs. Toss well

Mix garlic, lemon, zest and olive oil whip to mix well & toss with salad

Add salt & pepper to taste, toss to mix evenly. At this point serve or chill at 41°F until needed.

If you want to serve this as a meal you may add 1/4 to 1/3 cup per person of firm diced tofu, chicken, turkey, beef or pork.

Per Serving (excluding unknown items): 91 Calories; 6g Fat (58.0% calories from fat); 2g Protein; 8g Carbohydrate; 3g Dietary Fiber; 0mg Cholesterol; 189mg Sodium. Exchanges: 0 Grain(Starch); 0 Lean Meat; 1 1/2 Vegetable; 0 Fruit; 1Fat.

Crunchy Oven Fries

Whether you call them French fries or Cottage fries, these potatoes are heartwarming and comfort food at its best

Yield: 4 Cups

Preparation Time: 1 hour

Ingredients

1/2 Cup Grated Parmesan Cheese, divided in half
1 Teaspoon cayenne pepper, or to taste
2 Each egg
1 Tablespoon milk
1 Cup flour
1 Teaspoon Black Pepper
4 Cups French Fries, frozen

Servings: 8

Method

Mix Parmesan, cayenne and flour in a shallow bowl. In a second bowl whisk together egg and milk.

Dip frozen potatoes in egg-milk mixture then in season flour mixture, shaking excess flour.

Place on a foil lined baking sheet that has been lightly sprayed with non-stick cooking spray. Bake at 450ºF for 15 minutes or until fries are crisp and golden brown.

Per Serving (excluding unknown items): 462 Calories; 20g Fat (40.2% calories from fat); 10g Protein; 58g Carbohydrate;5g Dietary Fiber; 57mg Cholesterol; 346mg Sodium. Exchanges: 4 Grain(Starch); 1/2 Lean Meat; 0 Non-Fat Milk; 4 Fat.

Eggplant Paisana

A recipe from my mother's book Cociando en San Germán. Eggplant is my favorite vegetable. Try this one and it will be your favorite too.

Ingredients	Preparation Time: 45 minutes
1 Each Eggplants, peeled, sliced in 1/2" slices *1 Cup Stewed Tomatoes, chopped with juice* *1 Tablespoon Parsley, fresh chopped or 1 teaspoon dried flakes* *1 Tablespoon Oregano, fresh chopped or 1 teaspoon ground* *1 Each Green Bell Pepper, deveined, chopped* *2 Teaspoons Garlic Powder* *1 Teaspoon Pepper* *1 Tablespoon Olive Oil* *Serving Ideas: 1- Serve over pasta or rice* *2- Grate a good Parmesan cheese on it before serving*	Method Peel eggplant and slice about 1/2 inch thick Add remaining ingredients and toss to mix including the juice of the tomatoes Heat olive oil in large 2" pan and add eggplant mixture Cover and simmer until eggplant and peppers are tender If needed add reduced sodium chicken broth 1 tablespoon at a time

Servings: 6

Per Serving (excluding unknown items): 64 Calories; 3g Fat (32.8% calories from fat); 2g Protein; 10g Carbohydrate; 3g Dietary Fiber; 0mg Cholesterol; 15mg Sodium. Exchanges: 0 Grain(Starch); 1 1/2 Vegetable; 1/2 Fat.

Garbanzo Tomato Chopped Salad

A high protein salad you can make a meal out. Perfect for lunch or a light dinner.

Yield: 8 Servings

Ingredients

2 Cups Roma Tomato, Chopped
1/4 Cup olive oil
2 Dashes pepper
2 Cloves garlic, minced fine or 2 teaspoons garlic powder
4 Cans garbanzo beans, 15-ounce cans drained & rinsed
1 Cup Chopped Olives, pitted, chopped
1 Tablespoon thyme, fresh, chopped; or 1 tablespoon of dry thyme
1/2 Cup balsamic vinegar
2 Tablespoons chives, fresh chopped or 1 Tbsp dry

Servings: 8

Preparation Time: 20 minutes

Method

Chop tomatoes then mix all ingredients in a bowl

Toss and refrigerate to develop flavors

Serve on a bed of lettuce

Per Serving (excluding unknown items): 461 Calories; 15g Fat (28.4% calories from fat); 20g Protein; 66g Carbohydrate;19g Dietary Fiber; 0mg Cholesterol; 202mg Sodium. Exchanges: 4 Grain(Starch); 1 Lean Meat; 1/2 Vegetable; 0 Fruit; 2 1/2 Fat.

Gazpacho Salad

A twist on the classic Gazpacho - now you can eat it with a fork - one of my favorite summer salads perfect for a light lunch

Yield: 8 Cups

Preparation Time: 45 minutes

Ingredients

10 Each Ripe Tomatoes, large
2 Each Chopped Peeled Cucumber
1 Cup Chopped Green Bell Pepper
1/2 Cup finely chopped onion
1 Cup Romaine Lettuce
2 Cups Spinach Leaves, stems removed
1 Cup low fat bottled Italian dressing, make your own or use your favorite salad dressing
3 Cups mozzarella cheese, part skim milk, diced fine

Servings: 8

Method

Coarsely chop tomatoes, cucumbers, bell peppers and onions.

Combine all vegetables in a large salad bowl add Italian dressing and toss to coat well.

Serve the salad in large soup bowls and top with equal portions of diced or shredded mozzarella cheese

1 serving = 2 cups

Per Serving (excluding unknown items): 345 Calories; 28g Fat (69.8% calories from fat); 13g Protein; 14g Carbohydrate;3g Dietary Fiber; 38mg Cholesterol; 480mg Sodium. Exchanges: 1 ½ Lean Meat; 2 Vegetable; 0 Fruit; 4 ½ Fat.

Mediterranean Salad

A complete high protein meal with garbanzos

Yield: 8 Cups

Ingredients

1/2 Head Cauliflower, - about 2 pounds fresh, wash, core & chop
3 Large Cucumbers, peeled and chopped
4 Each Roma Tomato, quartered & seeded
1 Cup diced celery
2 2/3 Cans garbanzo beans, drained and rinsed (15 ounce each)
2/3 Cup flat leaf parsley, chopped
1/3 Cup cilantro, chopped
1/4 Cup chopped basil
1/3 Cup green onions, chopped
3 Cloves garlic, minced fine - or may use 1 tablespoon garlic powder instead
1 Cup Lemon Juice
2 Teaspoons lemon zest
1/2 Cup extra virgin olive oil
1 teaspoon kosher salt
1 Teaspoon pepper, black or white
1/2 Cup black olive, chopped

Serving Ideas: 1- Keeps refrigerated in a tightly covered container for up to 48 hours
2- Add variety and protein with diced meats, fish or tofu as desired.

Preparation Time: 30 minutes
Start to Finish Time: 30 minutes

Method

Cut cauliflower in half, core, wash and drain. Chop coarsely into flowerets.

Toss together with the garbanzos, cucumbers, tomatoes, celery & chopped herbs.

Mix garlic, lemon, zest and olive oil whip to mix well, pour over salad & toss to coat evenly

Add salt & pepper to taste, toss to mix evenly. At this point serve or chill at 41°F until needed.

Garnish with chopped black olives

Servings: 8

Per Serving (excluding unknown items): 420 Calories; 19g Fat (38.7% calories from fat); 15g Protein; 52g Carbohydrate; 15g Dietary Fiber; 0mg Cholesterol; 354mg Sodium. Exchanges: 2 1/2 Grain(Starch); 1/2 Lean Meat; 1 1/2 Vegetable; 0 Fruit; 3 1/2 Fat.

Spicy Beans

A protein packed side dish high in fiber, vitamins and minerals. Served over rice it's a hearty meal; add a salad or cooked vegetable to complete

1) For faster cooking cook in a pressure cooker or InstantPot on high pressure

2)To make in a slow cooker extend cooking time to 8 - 9 hours and plan to add more liquid halfway through cooking time

Yield: 6 cups

Preparation Time: 5 hours

Ingredients

1 tablespoon vegetable oil, or may use olive oil
1 teaspoon salt, or to taste
1 teaspoon pepper, or to taste
1 cup chopped onion
1/2 cup chopped green bell pepper
1/2 cup celery, sliced
1/2 cup carrot slices, fresh sliced
1/3 cup diced tomatoes, fresh
1 pound Beans, 1 pound dry beans = 2 cups
3 quarts Water or Reduced Sodium Broth
2 each bay leaf, whole, remove before serving
1 tablespoon ground oregano
1 tablespoon cilantro leaves, whole, chopped
2 teaspoons ground cumin
1 teaspoon Cayenne, or to taste
1 teaspoon Chili powder, or to taste

Serving Ideas: 1- Add greens such as spinach or kale for a more nutritious dish
2- Great with sliced avocados on top
3- Serve with Faro or barley instead of rice for a nice change and more fiber
4- Make a double batch and freeze half for another meal. May keep frozen for up to 3 months

Method

Soak & drain the beans

Heat oil and add all the chopped vegetables and seasonings. Sauté until tender.

Add tomatoes with juice and sauté mixing well with the other vegetables

Add drained soaked beans and water or broth.

Bring to a rolling boil, lower to simmer and cook for about 4 hours until tender. If using canned beans cook for one hour to blend flavors.

Serve as a side dish, with corn tortillas or over rice

Servings: 8

Per Serving (excluding unknown items): 227 Calories; 3g Fat (10.7% calories from fat); 13g Protein; 39g Carbohydrate; 15g Dietary Fiber; 0mg Cholesterol; 289mg Sodium. Exchanges: 2 1/2 Grain (Starch); 1 Lean Meat; 1/2 Vegetable; ½ Fat.

Spicy Jícama Salad

A spicy crunchy vegetable & fruit combination with a tangy dressing

Yield: 12 Cups

Ingredients

3 Pounds Jícama, peeled, cut in strips (small)
1 1/2 Cups orange juice
1/2 Cup lime juice, or may use lemon
1/2 Teaspoon salt, optional to enhance flavors
1 Teaspoon Black Pepper
1 Tablespoon Chili Powder
1 Tablespoon olive oil, 1/2" cubes
2 Each Apples, cored, sliced
2 Cups berries, any type, if strawberries cut into quarters
1 Cup cilantro, chopped - or may use any type of parsley or substitute dry flakes
12 Each romaine lettuce leaves
2 Tablespoons Green Onions, chopped and blanched
Serving Ideas: 1- Keeps in a tightly covered container for up to 48 hours
2- Serve it with a cup of hearty high protein soup for a complete meal

Preparation Time: 30 minutes
Start to Finish Time: 45 minutes
Method

Combine sliced (julienne) jícama and juices. Toss. Cover and chill for at least a half hour.

When ready to use add salt, pepper, oil, fruits, cilantro & chili powder and toss to mix and coat all fruits and jicama well.

Tear or chop Romaine leaves and toss with the chopped green onions. Scoop equal portions into the serving plates and serve the jícama salad on top

If desired drizzle extra dressing

Servings: 12

Per Serving (excluding unknown items): 98 Calories; 2g Fat (14.4% calories from fat); 2g Protein; 21g Carbohydrate; 7g Dietary Fiber; 0mg Cholesterol; 106mg Sodium. Exchanges: 1/2 Grain(Starch); 0 Lean Meat; 0 Vegetable; 1/2 Fruit; 0 Fat.

Spicy Sweet Potato Fries

Low fat, easy and nutritious as a snack or side dish

Yield: 1 Quart

Ingredients

4 Each sweet potato, small, scrubbed with skin up cut into 3X1 inch strips 0 cut lengthwise
1 Tablespoon vegetable oil
1 Teaspoon Cayenne Pepper
1 Teaspoon Coarse Salt
1 Teaspoon Paprika

Servings: 8

Preparation Time: 45 minutes

Method

Preheat oven to 450°F.

In a large bowl mix oil and cayenne pepper

Add sliced sweet potato strips & toss to coat well. Drain in colander or slotted spoon if too wet.

Grease baking sheet or line with parchment paper or foil with shiny side up. Spread drained strips on baking sheet and bake for 15 minutes

With a spatula turn strips to brown and toast evenly. Bake for 15 minutes.

Remove from oven and sprinkle with salt and paprika on both sides.

Per Serving (excluding unknown items): 85 Calories; 2g Fat (20.5% calories from fat); 1g Protein; 16g Carbohydrate; 2g Dietary Fiber; 0mg Cholesterol; 244mg Sodium. Exchanges: 1 Grain Starch); 0 Lean Meat; 1/2 Fat.

Sauces
Seasonings
& Soups

Ajilimójili

An all-purpose sauce originating in Puerto Rico and my secret ingredient for fish. Don't let this tongue twister hold you back. make it and love it. Just say A-HE-EE-LEE-MOHILI.

Yield: 2 cups

Preparation Time: 25 minutes

Ingredients

4 Cups cilantro, stemmed & chopped fine
2 Cups chives, chopped
1/2 Cup chopped garlic, or may use garlic paste if available
4 Cloves Garlic, peeled, leave whole
1 Cup balsamic vinegar
6 Each basil leaves
1 Cup rosemary, chopped or use 1 cup dry rosemary
1/2 Cup oregano, dry
1/2 Cup scallions, chopped
2 Cups Parmesan cheese
1 Teaspoon pepper, more or less to taste
6 Each Peppercorns, use whole
1 Teaspoon salt, more or less to taste
Serving Ideas: 1-Use to baste meats while cooking. If using as a basting sauce do not salt meats beforehand
2-Delicious added to meats on the side
3-Great when used as a salad dressing or for dipping crusty bread in
4-Toss with cooked pasta and serve with extra Parmesan cheese or cooked vegetables
5-Variations: add chopped olives or capers to mixture
6-Continue to add olive oil until solids are all used up

Method

After removing the stems, chop all ingredients except the olive oil together in a food processor or blender

Scrape into a glass jar and pour enough olive oil to cover. Stir to mix

Add the whole garlic cloves and peppercorns

Store in a glass jar with tight fitting lid.

Best when allowed to stand for a few hours for flavors to blend.

Will keep at room temperature for up to a week. If refrigerated it will keep longer but oil will harden so will have to allow to return to room temperature before using

Servings: 16

Per Serving (excluding unknown items): 96 Calories; 4g Fat (34.6% calories from fat); 7g Protein; 11g Carbohydrate; 3gDietary Fiber; 8mg Cholesterol; 338mg Sodium. Exchanges: 1/2 Grain(Starch); 1/2 Lean Meat; 1/2 Vegetable; 0 Fruit; 1/2 Fat.

Alabama Cream Sauce

A white BBQ sauce like no other. It's fantastic on fish and great on any meat

Yield: 2 Cups

Preparation Time: 10 minutes

Ingredients

1 Cup Mayonnaise
1/2 Cup Buttermilk
2 Tablespoons Horseradish
2 Tablespoons Vinegar
1 Tablespoon Cayenne
1 Tablespoon Garlic Powder
1 Teaspoon Pepper
2 Teaspoons Sugar

Method

Mix all ingredients well, store at 41°F in a tightly covered jar for up to 3 months

Servings: 16

Per Serving (excluding unknown items): 108 Calories; 12g Fat (91.6% calories from fat); 1g Protein; 2g Carbohydrate; trace Dietary Fiber; 5mg Cholesterol; 89mg Sodium. Exchanges: 0 Grain(Starch); 0 Non-Fat Milk; 1 Fat; 0 Other Carbohydrates.

Black and White Bean Soup

A very nutritious soup mildly spicy and so good!

Yield: 5/8 ounce

Ingredients

1 Cup dried black beans, washed and picked over
1 Cup dried white beans, washed and picked over
2 Quarts water
1/4 Cup Olive Oil
1 Cup Chopped Onion
1 Cup Diced Carrot
1 Clove garlic, minced - or may use 2 TB garlic powder
1/3 Tablespoon salt, taste and adjust at end before serving
1/2 Cup Chopped Tomatoes, chopped
1 Each bay leaves, whole
3 Each canned chipotle chiles, drained whole - or may use dried chiles
1 Quart Reduced Sodium Chicken Broth, or substitute vegetable broth
Serving Ideas: 1- May use canned beans instead of dried.
2- 1 lb dried beans = 2 1/4 cups dried beans

Servings: 8

Method

Place the black and the white beans in a medium saucepan with the water and bring to a boil. Turn down heat and simmer for 30 to 45 minutes until soft. Let simmer covered stirring occasionally to avoid sticking to the bottom

Heat oil and sauté the diced onions and all of the carrots and cook over medium low heat until onions are lightly browned, about 15 minutes. Add the garlic and salt, stirring constantly, until the garlic aroma is released, 1 - 2 minutes. Do not scorch the garlic as it will turn bitter.

Mix sautéed vegetables mixture with black & white beans and stir to mix well. Add broth and reheat.

Remove bay leaves and chipotle before serving.

Serve with 1/4 lime slice and additional chopped green onion tops and cilantro for each bowl as garnish. May also garnish with tomatillo, pico de gallo or red salsa and a dollop of sour cream if desired.

Per Serving (excluding unknown items): 254 Calories; 7g Fat (25.6% calories from fat); 13g Protein; 36g Carbohydrate;9g Dietary Fiber; 0mg Cholesterol; 610mg Sodium. Exchanges: 2 Grain(Starch); 1/2 Lean Meat; 1 Vegetable; 1 1/2 Fat.

Corn & Pepper Relish

Use on fish, pork or beef. Stores well for a week

1/4 Cup Olive Oil *1/2 Cup Diced Red Bell Pepper* *1/2 Cup Diced Green Bell Pepper* *2 Cups Whole Kernel Corn, Frozen* *1/2 Cup Diced Red Onion* *2 Cloves Garlic, crushed* *1/4 Cup Rum* *1/2 Cup Cream of Coconut* *1 Tablespoon Honey or Brown Sugar*	In a large skillet heat oil, add frozen corn and toss until golden brown on the edges Add onion, garlic and peppers, and continue to stir to blend flavors Add coconut cream, rum and honey or brown sugar and stir to mix. Simmer for 5 minutes Add salt and pepper to taste mixing well.

Per Serving (excluding unknown items): 1414 Calories; 77g Fat (50.9% calories from fat); 13g Protein; 155g Carbohydrate; 12g Dietary Fiber; 0mg Cholesterol; 77mg Sodium. Exchanges: 4 1/2 Grain(Starch); 3 Vegetable; 14 1/2 Fat; 4 1/2 Other Carbohydrates.

Crème Fraiche

Just a fancy word for a homemade sour cream.

Yield: 2 Cups
Ingredients
2 Cups Milk
2 Tablespoons Buttermilk
Servings: 8

Preparation Time: 15 minutes
Start to Finish Time: 4 hours
Method

In a clean jar mix the milk and buttermilk and stir gently to mix

If in a rush leave out at room temperature of about 72°F for 2 - 4 hours. If it's very hot it's best to place in the refrigerator for 8 hours

Keeps in tightly sealed glass container for 10 days

Per Serving (excluding unknown items): 39 Calories; 2g Fat (47.4% calories from fat); 2g Protein; 3g Carbohydrate; 0g Dietary Fiber; 8mg Cholesterol; 34mg Sodium. Exchanges: 1/2 Non-Fat Milk; 1/2 Fat.

Golden Winter Squash Soup

Take advantage of squash season and make this easy creamy soup. Use any type of squash.

Yield: 2 Quarts

Ingredients

2 Pounds winter squash, 4 cups diced
1/2 Cup onions, chopped
2 Cloves garlic, chopped
1 Each chili pepper, split lengthwise, seeded
1 1/2 Quarts Reduced Sodium Chicken Broth
1/2 Teaspoon Salt
1 Teaspoon pepper
1 Inch ginger, split lengthwise
1/2 Teaspoon turmeric, more or less to taste
1/2 Cup Half and Half
2 Teaspoons Ground Nutmeg, more or less to taste

Servings: 8

Preparation Time: 1 hour

Method

In a large soup pot or InstantPot mix all ingredients together and simmer until squash is tender.

Cool soup slightly for safety and mash the squash using an immersion blender

Add half and half, stir to mix and reheat to simmer. Don't boil it, the half and half will curdle

Add ground nutmeg before serving and stir to mix

Per Serving (excluding unknown items): 83 Calories; 2g Fat (23.1% calories from fat); 4g Protein; 13g Carbohydrate; 2g Dietary Fiber; 6mg Cholesterol; 550mg Sodium. Exchanges: 1/2 Grain(Starch); 1/2 Vegetable; 0 Non-Fat Milk; 1/2 Fat.

Hearty Gazpacho

A delicious cold soup for any time of the year. Perfect for summer picnics and BBQ

Yield: 1/2 Gallon

Preparation Time: 30 minutes

Ingredients

2 Each cucumber, peeled and diced
2 Each red and green bell pepper, seeded and diced
5 Each Roma tomatoes, or plum tomatoes, seeded, diced
1 Can Garbanzo Beans, drained & rinsed
1/2 Each red onion, chopped fine
4 Each Garlic Cloves, crushed
1 1/4 Quarts V-8® Vegetable Juice, No Added Salt, 2/23 oz cans
1/8 Cup white vinegar
1/8 Cup lemon juice
1/4 Cup olive oil
1/2 Teaspoon Kosher salt
2 Teaspoons black pepper
1 Teaspoon cayenne pepper, Optional or more or less to taste
2 Dashes Hot Sauce, I prefer Tabasco brand

Serving Ideas: 1-This is the perfect cold soup to take on a picnic. Pack in wide mouth thermos or tightly covered serving bowl to carry and keep refrigerated
2-Be sure to have extra hot sauce for those like very spicy foods
3-For a garnish try plain yogurt, chopped scallions or green onion tops, parsley or cilantro

Suggested Wine: dry red

Method

Chop or dice all vegetables - the size is up to you but the smaller the better results

In a large bowl whisk crushed garlic, olive oil, vinegar, lemon juice and salt and both peppers and toss with the chopped vegetables to coat well; let stand while getting the next ingredients ready

Pour vegetable juice over marinated vegetables and stir to mix well. Cover tightly and refrigerate overnight or for up to 32 hours. The longer it sits the more flavors develop but make sure temperature remains at 41°F

Serve in individual bowls or mugs making sure to get enough of each of the vegetables in each

Serve ice cold for the best taste with a drizzle of olive oil and a squeeze of lemon before serving

Servings: 8

Per Serving (excluding unknown items): 228 Calories; 9g Fat (33.0% calories from fat); 8g Protein; 32g Carbohydrate; 8g Dietary Fiber; 7mg Cholesterol; 172mg Sodium. Exchanges: 1 Grain(Starch); 1/2 Lean Meat; 3 Vegetable; 0 Fruit; 1 ½ Fat; 0 Other Carbohydrates.

Lemon-honey Salad Dressing

A lower fat & sugar version of a Paula Deen original

Yield: 2 Cups

Ingredients

1 1/2 Cups fresh lemon juice
1/2 Cup olive oil
1/3 Cup honey
8 Cloves garlic, diced or crushed, or 1 Tbsp garlic powder
2 Sprigs Fresh Thyme, needles removed & chopped fine
1/4 Cup Dijon Mustard
1/8 Teaspoon coarse salt
1 Teaspoon pepper

Servings: 16

Preparation Time: 15 minutes

Method

In a glass jar with a tight lid combine lemon juice, oil, honey, garlic & Dijon. Shake vigorously

Taste and add a dash of each Kosher salt and pepper. If too sour for your taste may add more honey.

Shake again; if not used immediately refrigerate up to a week

May also use a blender to mix into an emulsion or mix with wire whisk in a bowl if using garlic powder instead of garlic

Portion to taste over vegetable or fruit salads.

Keep refrigerated in sealed glass jar for up to 2 weeks.

Per Serving (excluding unknown items): 92 Calories; 7g Fat (63.3% calories from fat); trace Protein; 9g Carbohydrate; trace Dietary Fiber; 0mg Cholesterol; 62mg Sodium. Exchanges: 0 Grain(Starch); 0 Lean Meat; 0 Vegetable; 0 Fruit; 1 1/2 Fat; 1/2 Other Carbohydrates.

Mexican Style Seasoning

An easy, salt & preservative free Mexican style seasoning. This is my 'go to' seasoning for just about everything I cook these days. Use as a seasoning for any appropriate food

Yield: 3/4 cup

Ingredients

3 tablespoons chili powder
1 tablespoon cumin, ground
2 teaspoons paprika , smoked
2 teaspoons oregano, ground
1 teaspoon red pepper flakes, crush or grind
1/2 teaspoon pepper
1 teaspoon garlic powder
1/2 teaspoon onion powder

Serving Ideas: 1- Mix 2 - 3 tablespoons with 1/2 teaspoon cornstarch and 1 cup water for 1# ground or diced meat
2- Rub on whole meats or chickens and let sit for at least 1 hour before cooking
3- For a dip or sauce: Mix 3 tablespoons with 2 cups sour cream or yogurt

Preparation Time: 10 minutes

Method

Measure ingredients in a mason or other glass jar. Cover and shake jar to mix all ingredients well to combine.

Stores indefinitely stored with your other seasonings.

Servings: 6

Per Serving (excluding unknown items): 20 Calories; 1g Fat (32.6% calories from fat); 1g Protein; 3g Carbohydrate; 2g Dietary Fiber; 0mg Cholesterol; 40mg Sodium. Exchanges: 0 Grain(Starch); 0 Lean Meat; 0 Fat.

Mushroom Wild Rice Soup

This is also a perfect soup to make in the InstantPot cooker and then you don't have to watch it much My most favorite soup; a holiday tradition in my family but I make it often as it makes a perfect late dinner meal. Rich, savory and satisfying this hearty soup has been a tradition in our family for any occasion.

Yield: 8 Cups

Ingredients

2 Quarts Reduced Sodium Chicken Broth
3 Pounds Mushrooms
1/4 Cup Olive Oil
5 Each Garlic Cloves, diced - or substitute 1 tablespoon garlic powder
1 Cup Green Onions, sliced
1/4 Teaspoon Salt
1 Teaspoon Pepper
1 Cup Half and Half
2 Cups Skim Milk
1 Cup Wild Rice

Servings: 8

Preparation Time: 2 hours

Method

In a soup pot heat olive oil and add onions, and salt; sauté about 10 minutes stirring to prevent scorching onions

Coarsely chop mushrooms and add to pot with 2 tablespoons of butter. Continue sautéing until both mushrooms and onions are golden brown then lower heat and add garlic and pepper. Stir to mix and cover for 5 minutes

Add broth, cover and simmer for 30 minutes to blend flavors.

When mushrooms are tender add wild rice. Quickly bring to a boil on high heat then lower heat , cover and simmer for 1 hour or until rice cooks all the way through and grains burst open.

Remove from heat and add milk and half and half. Adjust seasonings. Reheat again at a low simmer for 5 - 10 minutes without boiling to prevent curdling

Garnish with additional sliced green onions and a few small raw mushroom caps for crunch.

Per Serving (excluding unknown items): 250 Calories; 11g Fat (38.6% calories from fat); 12g Protein; 29g Carbohydrate; 4g Dietary Fiber; 12mg Cholesterol; 660mg Sodium. Exchanges: 1 Grain(Starch); 2 Vegetable; 1/2 Non-Fat Milk; 2 Fat.

My Favorite Chicken Soup

Good enough for a satisfying meal. My favorite chicken soup and it's not my mother's soup
1- A whole chicken yields enough boned meat for a second meal such as chicken salad or pot pie.
2- Don't try to reuse the strained ingredients; they're colorless, mushy and flavorless.
3- During preparation the broth and chicken are safe while working for under two hours. If you take longer be sure to keep both broth and chicken either cool at below 41°F or hot above 135°F for safety.
4- If more liquid is needed use reduced or low sodium chicken broth.
5- Once vegetables, potatoes, rice/noodles cook, add chicken meat & simmer to 165°F for 15 to 20 seconds. Chicken meat becomes stringy when overcooked or boiled.

Yield: 1 Gallon

Preparation Time: 3 hours

Ingredients

1 Whole Chicken, 3-5#
1 Gallon Water
1 Each Onion, peeled and quartered
1 Each Ham Hock, fat removed
6 Each Garlic Cloves, peeled & crushed
2 Inch Ginger Root Slices, peeled
1 Teaspoon Salt
2 Teaspoons Pepper
3 Stalks Celery, cut in 1" slices
4 Large Carrots, cut in 1" slices
1 Bunch Italian Parsley
1/4 Cup Fresh Oregano, or 2 Tbsp dry flakes
1 Large Bay Leaf
2 Each Potatoes, peeled and cubed
1 Tablespoon Soy Sauce, Low Sodium, good quality Chinese
Serving Ideas: 1- Vegetables: carrots, spinach, kale, green beans, peas, celery
2- Potatoes: If using potatoes add after the vegetables and do not overcook or they will fall apart.
3- Rice or Noodles: Limit amount added as they will absorb a lot of liquid and if held overnight keep absorbing moisture soaking most of the broth becoming thick and mushy.

Method

In a deep soup pot add tap water, quartered chicken or chicken pieces, vegetables, herbs & spices Bring to a short boil, turn down, simmer for 1 to 2 hours.

Let soup cool enough to handle, strain broth and set aside.

Bone chicken, remove & discard skin and discard vegetables, ham, ginger & bay leaf.

Bone chicken & remove skin. A whole chicken yields enough boned meat for a second meal such as chicken salad or pot pie.

Add your choice of freshly chopped vegetables as desired and your choice of diced potatoes, rice or pasta. Simmer until done.

Adjust seasonings. Finish soup with 1 tablespoon of soy sauce. Stir and serve.

Servings: 12

Per Serving (excluding unknown items): 328 Calories; 21g Fat (58.9% calories from fat); 25g Protein; 9g Carbohydrate;2g Dietary Fiber; 122mg Cholesterol; 351mg Sodium. Exchanges: 1/2 Grain(Starch); 3 Lean Meat; 1 Vegetable; 2 Fat.

Pizzazz Pumpkin Soup

A savory, spicy pumpkin soup light in calories packed with nutritious vitamins.

Ingredients

1 Tablespoon Butter
2 Tablespoons Olive Oil
1/3 Cup Chopped Onion
1/2 Cup Chopped Celery
4 Cloves Chopped Garlic
1/4 Cup Chopped Cilantro
1 Each Bay Leaf, chopped
1/2 Teaspoon Ground Thyme
2 Tablespoons Chili Powder, New Mexico is best for the smoky taste
1 Tablespoon Tabasco Sauce, optional
6 Cups Reduced Sodium Chicken Broth
1 Can Pumpkin Purée, 15 oz. can unsweetened
1 1/2 Cups Half and Half, or substitute milk
1 Teaspoon Ground Nutmeg
Serving Ideas: Garnish the soup with chopped herbs, sour cream, a drizzle of olive oil, diced ham, scallions or onions
For even more pizzazz add cayenne.
To reduce fat & increase protein use milk instead of half & half

Method

Heat butter & oil and add chopped vegetables (next 5 ingredients). Sauté until onion is clear and vegetables tender

Season with salt & pepper, stir and sauté for a minute longer

Stir in flour, spices & hot sauce; stir well until flour absorbs all the liquid and starts to thicken

Stir in broth, bring to simmer

Add pumpkin purée & stir to avoid or remove lumps until soup is thickened

Add half & half or milk, stir constantly and bring to a light simmer

Top with a shake or two of nutmeg before serving and garnish with additional chopped cilantro

Servings: 8

Per Serving (excluding unknown items): 133 Calories; 11g Fat (69.0% calories from fat); 4g Protein; 7g Carbohydrate; 2g Dietary Fiber; 21mg Cholesterol; 474mg Sodium. Exchanges: 0 Grain (Starch); 1 Vegetable; 0 Non-Fat Milk; 2 Fat.

Spicy Apple Cranberry Relish

A different relish to use with meats, or even spoon in soups - an excellent complement to Pizazz Pumpkin Soup

Ingredients	Method
1 Each Large Apple, cored & chopped with peel *1/4 Each Red Onion, diced* *1/4 Cup Lime Juice* *1/2 Cup Dried Cranberries* *1 Teaspoon Chili Powder* *2 Teaspoons Honey* *1/2 Teaspoon Cinnamon* *1/4 Teaspoon Cayenne* **Servings: 6**	Combine chopped apple, onion, lime juice, cranberries, chili powder, cayenne, honey & cinnamon Toss to coat all ingredients Cover and store in refrigerator for at least one hour before using

Per Serving (excluding unknown items): 36 Calories; trace Fat (5.2% calories from fat); trace Protein; 9g Carbohydrate;1g Dietary Fiber; 0mg Cholesterol; 5mg Sodium. Exchanges: 0 Grain (Starch); 0 Vegetable; 1/2 Fruit; 0 Fat; 0 Other Carbohydrates.

Spicy Sauce

A delicious sauce to use on meats - use sparingly as it's very high in sodium

Yield: 3 Cups

Preparation Time: 15 minutes

Ingredients

8 Cloves garlic, chopped fine
1 Cup Dark Brown Sugar
1 Cup honey
1 Cup Low Sodium Soy Sauce
1/2 Cup Worcestershire sauce
1 Tablespoon ground ginger
1 Teaspoon ground cinnamon
2 Teaspoons cayenne pepper
1/2 Cup ketchup, optional if a sweeter sauce is desired
Serving Ideas: 1-Use to baste meats while cooking. If using as a basting sauce do not salt meats beforehand
2-Delicious added to meats on the side

Method

Measure all ingredients in a glass jar.

Cover and shake well to mix

Store refrigerated at 41°F for up to 30 days

Servings: 16

Per Serving (excluding unknown items): 144 Calories; trace Fat (0.6% calories from fat); 1g Protein; 37g Carbohydrate; trace Dietary Fiber; 0mg Cholesterol; 769mg Sodium. Exchanges: 0 Grain(Starch); 1/2 Vegetable; 0 Fat; 2 1/2 Other Carbohydrates.

Whipped Brandy Caramel Sauce

Sweet topping for any desert. Instead of Brandy you can use any other liquor, or a citrus juice such as orange, Yuzu or lemon. This is a great compliment to the Pumpkin Bread Pudding or any other bread pudding that is not too sweet.

Yield: 2 cups

Preparation Time: 20 minutes

Ingredients

1 1/2 cups packed dark brown sugar
1/2 cup butter, unsalted
1 cup whipped cream, measure 1 cup after whipping
cup brandy, c choose a good brand you would want to drink
Serving Ideas: 1 - Serve over cakes, ice creams, puddings.
2- Try as a topping on French Toast or Waffles for a quick dessert using "leftovers" from breakfast
Suggested Wine: Brandy

Servings: 16

Method

Melt butter in small saucepan.

Add brown sugar and stir until sugar is mixed then add 1/2 cup whipping cream and whisk until the mixture is smooth. Give it a good whisk to remove all lumps and smooth the mixture.

Cool slightly and add brandy, whisking until mixed well.

Whip whipping cream until stiff being careful not to separate the whey and turn it to butter.

Fold the caramel mixture into the whipped cream gently, then stir a few times to ensure it's well mixed.

Refrigerate until use and stir again before serving as the caramel separates after a few hours.

This freezes well and can be made in advance, storing in zip lock bags until needed.

Per Serving (excluding unknown items): 154 Calories; 9g Fat (48.3% calories from fat); trace Protein; 20g Carbohydrate;0g Dietary Fiber; 26mg Cholesterol; 69mg Sodium. Exchanges: 0 Non-Fat Milk; 1 1/2 Fat; 1 1/2 Other Carbohydrates.

Recipes Index

Recipes Index

Recipes Index

I'm just someone who likes cooking and for whom sharing food is a form of expression.

Maya Angelou

Made in United States
Orlando, FL
04 November 2026

90202056R00055